SpringerBriefs in Electrical and Computer Engineering

For further volumes:
http://www.springer.com/series/10059

Liana Stanescu • Dumitru Dan Burdescu
Marius Brezovan • Cristian Gabriel Mihai

Creating New Medical Ontologies for Image Annotation

A Case Study

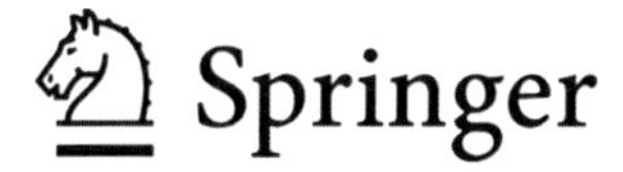

Liana Stanescu
Department of Software Engineering
University of Craiova
Craiova 200585, Romania
stanescu@software.ucv.ro

Dumitru Dan Burdescu
Department of Software Engineering
University of Craiova
Craiova 200585, Romania
burdescu_dumitru@software.ucv.ro

Marius Brezovan
Department of Software Engineering
University of Craiova
Craiova 200585, Romania
mbrezovan@software.ucv.ro

Cristian Gabriel Mihai
Department of Software Engineering
University of Craiova
Craiova 200585, Romania
mihai_gabriel@software.ucv.ro

ISSN 2191-8112 e-ISSN 2191-8120
ISBN 978-1-4614-1908-2 e-ISBN 978-1-4614-1909-9
DOI 10.1007/978-1-4614-1909-9
Springer New York Dordrecht Heidelberg London

Library of Congress Control Number: 2011943747

Printed on acid-free paper

Springer is part of Springer Science+Business Media (www.springer.com)

Preface

Advances in medical technology generate huge amounts of nontextual information (e.g., images) along with more familiar textual one. The image is one of the most important tools in medicine since it provides a method for diagnosis, monitoring, and disease management of patients with the advantage of being a very fast noninvasive procedure.

As new image acquisition devices are constantly being developed, to increase efficiency and produce more accurate information, and data storage capacity increases, a steady growth of the number of medical images produced can be easily inferred. With such an exponential increase of medical data in digital libraries, it is becoming more and more difficult to execute certain analysis on search and information retrieval-related tasks.

Such problems can be tackled by representing the available information using languages such as DAML+OIL and OWL, which benefit from their underlying description logic foundation. Recently, there has been lot of discussion about semantically enriched information systems, especially about using ontologies for modeling data. Ontologies have the potential of modeling information in a way that they can capture the meaning of the content by using expressive knowledge representation formalisms, such as description logics, and therefore achieve good information retrieval results.

In this book, we outline our experience of building a semantically system by accommodating image annotation and retrieval services around an ontology for medical images used in digestive diseases. Our approach is based on the assumptions that, given images from digestive diseases, expressing all the desired features using domain knowledge is feasible, and manually marking up and annotating the regions of interest is practical. In addition, by developing an automatic annotation system, representing and reasoning about medical images are performed with a reasonable complexity in a given querying context.

This book is mainly intended for scientists and engineers who are engaged in research and development of visual information retrieval techniques, especially for medical color images from the area of digestive diseases, and who want to move from content-based visual information retrieval to semantic-based visual information retrieval.

The objective of this book is to review and survey new research and development in intelligent visual information retrieval technologies, and to present a system for semantic-based visual information retrieval in collections of medical images that aims to reduce the "semantic gap" in image understanding.

The book includes seven chapters that cover several distinctive research fields in visual information retrieval ranging between content-based to semantic-based visual retrieval and from low-level to high-level image features. They also provide many state-of-the-art advancements and achievements in filling the semantic gap.

The book is structured in four distinct sections. The first part gives an overview of the content-based image retrieval, and it contains only the Chap. 2. The second part deals with the problem of image segmentation that is necessary for identifying visual objects from images, and it contains the Chap. 3. The third part looks of some aspects concerning image annotation by using ontologies, and it contains two chapters: Chaps. 4 and 5. The last part deals with the problem of semantic-based image retrieval, and it presents an object-oriented system for visual information retrieval from medical images, which uses both content-based and semantic-based visual searching.

Overall, the book contains several pictures and several dozen tables that offer a comprehensive image about the current advancements of semantic-based visual information retrieval.

Craiova, Romania

Liana Stanescu
Dumitru Dan Burdescu
Marius Brezovan
Cristian Gabriel Mihai

Contents

Chapter 1
Introduction

Medical images play a central role in patient diagnosis, therapy, surgical planning, medical reference, and medical training. With the advent of digital imaging modalities, as well as images digitized from conventional devices, collections of medical images are increasingly being held in digital form. Due to the large number of images without text information, content-based medical image retrieval has received increased attention.

Content-based visual information retrieval (CBVIR) has attracted many interests, from image engineering, computer vision, and database community. A large number of researches have been developed and have achieved plentiful and substantial results. Content-based image retrieval task could be described as a process for efficiently retrieving images from a collection by similarity. The retrieval relies on extracting the appropriate characteristic quantities describing the desired contents of images. Most CBVIR approaches rely on the low-level visual features of image and video, such as color, texture, and shape. Such techniques are called feature-based techniques in visual information retrieval. The second chapter of the book, "Content-Based Image Retrieval in Medical Images Databases," deals with the CBVIR approaches, presenting a general overview, an evaluation method of the CBVIR task.

Unfortunately, current methods of the CBVIR systems only focus on appearance-based similarity, that is, the appearance of the retrieved images is similar to that of a query image. There is little semantic information exploited. Among the few efforts which claim to exploit the semantic information, the semantic similarities are defined between different appearances of the same object. These kinds of semantic similarities represent the low-level semantic similarities, while and the similarities between different objects represent the high-level semantic similarities. The similarities between two images are the similarities between the objects contained by the two images.

As a consequence, a way to develop a semantic-based visual information retrieval (SBVIR) system consists in two steps: (1) to extract the visual objects from images and (2) to associate semantic information to each visual object. The first step can be

L. Stanescu et al., *Creating New Medical Ontologies for Image Annotation: A Case Study*, SpringerBriefs in Electrical and Computer Engineering,
DOI 10.1007/978-1-4614-1909-9_1,

achieved by using segmentation methods applied to images, while the second step can be achieved by using semantic annotation methods to the visual objects extracted from images.

Image segmentation techniques can be distinguished into two groups, region-based and contour-based approaches. Region-based segmentation methods can be broadly classified as either top-down (model-based) or bottom-up (visual feature-based) approaches. An important group of visual feature-based methods is represented by the graph-based segmentation methods, which attempt to search a certain structures in the associated edge-weighted graph constructed on the image pixels, such as minimum spanning tree or minimum cut. Other approaches to image segmentation consist of splitting and merging regions according to how well each region fulfills some uniformity criterion. Such methods use a measure of uniformity of a region. In contrast, other methods use a pairwise region comparison rather than applying a uniformity criterion to each individual region. The third chapter of the book, "Medical Images Segmentation," describes some graph-based color segmentation methods and an area-based evaluation framework of the performance of the segmentation algorithms.

The second step of the proposed SBIR system involves an annotation process of the visual objects extracted from images. It becomes increasingly expensive to manually annotate medical images. Consequently, automatic medical image annotation becomes important. We consider image annotation as a special classification problem, that is, classifying a given image into one of the predefined labels.

Automatic image annotation is the process of assigning meaningful words to an image, taking into account its content. This process is of great interest as it allows indexing, retrieving, and understanding of large collections of image data. There are two reasons that are making the image annotation a difficult task: the semantic gap, being hard to extract semantically meaningful entities using just low-level image features and the lack of correspondence between the keywords and image regions in the training data. Several interesting techniques have been proposed in the image annotation research field. Most of these techniques define a parametric or nonparametric model to capture the relationship between image features and keywords. The problem of image annotation is presented in the fifth chapter of the book, "Medical Images Annotation." In this chapter is presented an overview of the existing methods for the annotation task from several perspectives: unsupervised/supervised learning, parametric/nonparametric unsupervised learning models, or text/image based. An extension of the cross-media relevance model based on an object-oriented approach has been choosing for medical images annotation, and an evaluation of the annotation process and the experimental results are presented in the final part of the chapter.

The concepts used for annotation of visual objects are generally structured in hierarchies of concepts that form different ontologies. The notion of ontology is defined as an explicit specification of some conceptualization, while the conceptualization is defined as an intensional semantic structure that encodes the rules of constraining the structure of a part of reality. The goal of an ontology is to define some primitives and their associated semantics in some specified context. Ontologies have been established for knowledge sharing and are widely used as a means for conceptually structuring domains of interest. With the growing usage of ontologies, the problem of overlapping knowledge in a common domain occurs more often and becomes critical. Domain-specific ontologies are modeled by multiple authors in multiple settings. These ontologies lay the foundation for building new domain-specific ontologies in similar domains by assembling and extending multiple ontologies from repositories.

Ontologies are frequently used in medical domain, and for this reason several aspects related to the applicability of the ontology in this domain are presented. Existing ontologies are provided in formats that are not always easy to interpret and use. A high flexibility is obtained when an ontology is created from scratch using a custom approach. Because of this, in the fourth chapter of the book, "Ontologies," it is described a custom approach for obtaining an ontology using a medical source of information like MeSH. The content of an ontology needs to be stored in a specific format. The Topic Maps standard was proved to be an efficient mechanism that can be successfully used to represent the content of our ontology.

Image retrieval based on the semantic meaning of the images is currently being explored by many researchers. The five levels of semantics are considered to be the following (from weak semantics to strong semantics): free text, controlled vocabulary, taxonomy, thesaurus, and ontology. Automatic image annotation is the attempt to discover concepts and keywords that represent the image. This can be done by predicting concepts to which an object belongs. When a successful mapping between the visual perception and keyword is achieved, the image annotation can be indexed to reduce image search time. In the first parts of the sixth chapter of the book, "Semantic-Based Image Retrieval," there are presented four classes of methods toward semantic image retrieval: (1) automatic scene classification in whole images by statistically based techniques, (2) methods for learning and propagating labels assigned by human users, (3) automatic object classification using knowledge-based or statistical techniques, and (4) retrieval methods with relevance feedback during a retrieval session. Several approaches from these classes are presented and analyzed. The second part of this chapter proposes an efficient method called semantic-based image retrieval using cross-media relevance model (CMRM). CMRM allows two models for semantic-based image retrieval: probabilistic annotation-based cross-media relevance model (PACMRM) and direct-retrieval cross-media relevance model (DRCMRM). At the end of the chapter, experimental results made using the methods provided by the CMRM model for ranked image retrieval are presented.

The last chapter of the book, "Object Oriented Medical Annotation System," proposes and presents in detail an object-oriented medical annotation software system, called MASOO, for proving the means for evaluating the performance of the annotation or retrieval task. The annotation system contains two distinct modules, the client component and the server component, and it uses a db4o database. The system MASOO can be used for three distinct tasks: (1) automatic image annotation using the cross-media relevance model, (2) semantic-based image retrieval using two methods exposed by the CMRM model, and (3) content-based image retrieval based on color and texture features.

Chapter 2
Content-Based Image Retrieval in Medical Images Databases

2.1 Introduction

In the medical domain, in the diagnosis, treatment, and research processes, traditional alphanumerical information (patient personal data, diagnosis, results for the analysis, and investigations) and a large quantity of images are accumulated. The tendency is to digitalize the images. At present, a large variety of digital image modalities are used: film scanners, computed tomography (CT), positron emission tomography (PET), single positron emission computed tomography (SPECT), ultrasounds, magnetic resonance imaging (MRI), digital subtraction angiography (DSA), and magnetic source imaging (MSI) [1].

It is considered that the medical domains that produce the highest number of images are the cardiology and radiology. Also the endoscope images are produced in significant quantities. For example, the University Hospital of Geneva gathers more than 13,000 images daily, from more than 30 types of medical devices. Besides that, there are many other images stored on other media. But the largest volume of image data is produced in the hospitals from the United States where digital images represent 30% and the other 70% represent images acquired in conventional X-rays and digital luminescent radiography modalities. The X-ray films can be digitized with different tools [1].

The storage of medical images in digital format makes their transferring from one device to another an easy task and enhances the achieving and manipulation process, in a useful and novel way.

Medical image management plays now an important role in designing and implementing medical information systems. It is needed to introduce new methods for representation, manipulation, and search for multimedia information.

The modern technique to retrieve multimedia information considering attributes or characteristics extracted from multimedia information and finding multimedia objects that have these types of characteristics in common is called content-based retrieval.

L. Stanescu et al., *Creating New Medical Ontologies for Image Annotation: A Case Study*, SpringerBriefs in Electrical and Computer Engineering,
DOI 10.1007/978-1-4614-1909-9_2,

Content-based visual retrieval can be implemented, taking into consideration primitive visual characteristics (color, texture, shape), logical characteristics (object identity), or abstract characteristics (scene semantics). The easiest way for implementation is to use primitive characteristics as color, texture, and shape [2–4].

The objective of the content-based visual query is to search and retrieve in an efficient manner those images from the database that are most appropriate to the image considered by the user as query [4]. The content-based visual query differs from the usual query by the fact it implies the similarity search.

There are two forms of content-based visual query [4]:

- The K-nearest neighborhood query that retrieves the most appropriate K images with the query image
- Range query that retrieves all the images that respect a fixed limit of the similarity confronted by the query image.

The directions where content-based retrieval is needed in medical multimedia databases were fully specified. They are [5, 6]:

- Diagnostic aid—from the conversation with the doctors, the following situation appears frequently: the doctor visualizes a medical image, he/she cannot establish the diagnosis exactly, he/she is aware of the fact that he/she has seen something similar before but does not have the means to search for it in the database; the problem can be solved establishing that image as query image, and the content-based image query will provide the similar images from the database; it is very likely that among the retrieved images should be the searched image together with its diagnosis, observations, treatment; so the content-based image query can be directly used in the diagnosis process.
- Medical teaching—there is a series of applications for content-based visual query including other ways for access (text-based, hierarchical methods). Students can see the images in the database and the attached information in a simple and direct manner; they choose the query image, and they see the similar images; this method stimulates learning by comparing similar cases and their particularities or comparing similar cases with different diagnosis.
- Medical research—using content-based visual query in this area brings up similar advantages for medical teaching. It can be used, for example, for finding certain types of images to be included in a study, for finding misclassified images, etc.
- PACS and electronic records for patients—the integration of the content-based visual retrieval techniques and the simple text-based retrieval in PACS and the electronic patients' record might bring important benefits in clinical applications. The information that is stored in the image can be used together with the alphanumerical information.

2.2 Content-Based Image Retrieval Systems

There is in present a series of database management systems capable to manage different types of media. Many of these systems permit indexing and searching for multimedia information, taking into account only structured information, using traditional techniques. They work well only with short numeric and alphanumeric arrays. This includes traditional queries of the databases based on alphanumerical arrays. They cannot be used for multimedia information indexing and retrieval. That is why the researchers studied the possibility to create new systems that satisfy the high demands of the multimedia information.

An exception is Oracle Multimedia (formerly Oracle interMedia), a feature of Oracle Database that enables the efficient management and retrieval of image, audio, and video data. Oracle Multimedia has knowledge of the most popular multimedia formats and makes automate metadata extraction and basic image processing.

Most of the medical informatics systems use for multimedia medical databases management traditional database management servers (MySQL, MS SQL Server, Interbase, Oracle). There have been implemented alternative methods for content-based visual retrieval, taking into consideration different characteristics like color, texture, and shape.

For medical multimedia databases content-based query, it is generally used the method called QBE (Query by Example). It implies the selection of an image or a region as a query image (region). It can be also combined the simple text-based query with an image (region) query [5].

In general, the images are represented in the databases by automatically extracted visual features that are supposed to correspond to the visual image content or the way we perceive it. The features mainly used for image retrieval, are [5, 7]:

- Gray levels and color descriptors, in a local or global fashion
- Texture descriptors
- Shapes of segmented objects

Content-based retrieval has been investigated in few important projects. It can be mentioned the QBIC project from IBM [8, 9] and Virage, a commercial project for content-based retrieval [8]. Most of the projects are academically projects: Photobook system from MIT [8], MARS (Multimedia Analysis and Retrieval System) developed to the University of Illinois [8, 10], Chabot system for image retrieval [11], WebSEEk system, VisualSEEk, and SaFe implemented to the University of Columbia [8, 11–14]. Using higher-level information, such as segmented parts of the image for queries, was introduced by the Blobworld system [15].

A system that is available free of charge is the GNU Image Finding Tool (GIFT). Some systems are available as demonstration versions on the web such as Viper, WIPE, or Compass [5].

Generally, these systems have a similar architecture that includes: modules for medical characteristics extraction from images and their storage in the databases, modules for content-based retrieval, taking into consideration the extracted characteristics and the user interface [5].

Although the number of the medical informatics systems that implement efficiently the content-based retrieval process is high, it is used in practice only a small number of them. An example is IRMA project that brings important contributions in two research fields [16, 17]:

- Automated classification of radiographs based on global features with respect to imaging modality, direction, body region examined, and biological system under investigation.
- Identification of image features that are relevant for medical diagnosis. These features are derived from a priori classified and registered images.

The system can retrieve images that are similar to a query image, taking into consideration a selected set of features. The research was done on image data consists of radiographs, but will be extended on medical images from arbitrary modalities.

Another important CBIR system for the domain of HRCT (high-resolution computed tomography) images of the lung with emphysema-type diseases is ASSERT [18, 19]. It was developed at Purdue University in collaboration with the Department of Radiology at Indiana University and the School of Medicine at the University of Wisconsin. Because the symptoms of these diseases can drastically alter the appearance of the texture of the lung, can vary widely across patients and based on the severity of the disease, ASSERT system characterizes the images using low-level features like texture features computed from the co-occurrence matrix of the image. The retrieval is performed hierarchically. At the first level, the disease category of the query image is predicted. At the second level, the most similar images to the query image that belong to the predicted class are retrieved and displayed to the user.

Also, it must be mentioned the MedGIFT system, implemented to the University Hospital from Geneva [6]. It was developed to work together with CasImage, a radiological teaching file that has been used in daily routine for several years now. The system works with more than 60,000 images from more than 10,000 medical cases. The database is available on the intranet of the hospital, with a smaller database being publicly available via Internet and MIRC. The system contains modules for image feature extraction, feature indexing structures, and a communication interface called MRML (Multimedia Retrieval Markup Language).

MedGIFT uses techniques from text retrieval such as [6]:

- Frequency-based feature weights
- Inverted file indexing structures
- Relevance feedback mechanisms

Four feature groups represent the image content [6]:

- Local and global texture features based on responses of Gabor filters
- Color/grayscale characteristics on a global image scale and locally within image regions

The interface allows for an easy integration into applications such as [6]:

- Teaching file
- Document management systems
- Tools for diagnostic aid

There are a large variety of applications and studies of content-based visual retrieval that takes into consideration the images from different medical departments. Most of them use databases with images produced in radiology departments, but there are many other departments where this type of algorithms have been implemented. Few of these categories of images are [5]:

- Dermatologic images.
- Cytological specimens.
- Pathology images have often been proposed for content-based access as the color and texture properties can relatively easy be identified; the pathologist can use a CBIR system instead of books when searching for reference cases.
- Histopathology images.
- Histology images.
- Cardiology.
- Within the radiology department, mammography is one of the most frequent application areas.
- Ultrasound images of the breast and other ultrasound images.
- High-resolution computed tomography (HRCT) scans of the lung.
- Endoscopic images from digestive area.

It must be mentioned that all these applications and studies have been implemented using multimedia medical databases that are extremely varied in size and quality [5]. It starts from tens or hundreds, ending with thousands. The results of these studies are more solid as the dimension of the database is higher and if the images are acquired from the investigation and diagnosis process of the patients. One of the biggest databases used in studies use only simulated images. Although these simulated images are easy and cheap to obtain, their use for any qualitative assessments is more than questionable [5].

Databases that have been used in content-based visual retrieval study have only few tens or hundreds of medical images, and it is considered to be too small for delivering any statistically significant measurements [5].

2.3 Content-Based Image Query on Color and Texture Features

The objective of the content-based visual query is to search and retrieve in an efficient manner those images from the database that are most appropriate to the image considered by the user as query. The content-based visual query differs from the usual query by the fact that it implies the similitude search. Visual elements such as color, texture, shape that directly describe the visual content, and also high-level concepts (e.g., the significance of the objects) are used for retrieving images with a similar content from the database [2].

The usage of the color and texture features in content-based image query will lead to better results in some diseases. There are some diseases that are characterized by the change of the color and the texture of the affected tissue, for example, ulcer, colitis, esophagitis, polyps, ulcer, and ulcerous tumor.

In content-based visual query on color feature (the color is the visual feature immediately perceived on an image), the used color space and the level of quantization, meaning the maximum number of colors, are of great importance. The color histograms represent the traditional method of describing the color properties of the images. They have the advantages of easy computation and up to a certain point are insensitive to camera rotating, zooming, and changes in image resolution [7]. The solution of representing the color information extracted from images using HSV color space, quantized to 166 colors, was chosen. It was proved that the HSV color system has the following properties [7]: it is close to the human perception of colors, it is intuitive, and it is invariant to illumination intensity and camera direction.

The operation of color quantization is needed in order to reduce the number of colors used in content-based visual query from millions to tens. The chosen solution was proposed by J. R. Smith, namely, the quantization of the HSV space to 166 colors [4, 20]. Because the hues represent the most important color feature, a most refined quantization is necessary. In the circle that represents the color, the primary colors, red, green, and blue, are separated by 120 degrees. A circular quantization with a 20-degree step sufficiently separates the colors, such that the primary colors and yellow, magenta, and cyan colors are each represented by three subdivisions. The saturation and the value are each quantized to three levels. This quantization produces 18 hues, three saturations, three values, and four grays, in total 166 distinct colors in the HSV color space. The experimental studies made both on images from nature and medical images have proven that choosing the HSV color space, quantized to 166 colors, is one of the best choices in order to have a content-based visual query process of good quality [20]. The 166 colors histogram will be used in the content-based visual query process.

Together with color, texture is a powerful characteristic of an image, existent in nature and medical images, where a disease can be indicated by changes in the color and texture of a tissue. There are many techniques used for texture extraction, but there is not a certain method that can be considered the most appropriate, this depending on the application and the type of images taken into account [2]. One of the most representative methods for texture detection is the method that uses co-occurrence matrices [2]. For an image $f(x, y)$, the co-occurrence matrix $hd\phi\ (i, j)$ is defined so that each entry (i, j) is equal to the number of times for that $f(x_1, y_1) = i$ and $f(x_2, y_2) = j$, where $(x_2, y_2) = (x_1, y_1) + (d\cos\phi, d\sin\phi)$. In the case of color images, one matrix is computed for each of the three channels (R, G, B). This leads to three quadratic matrices of dimension equal to the number of the color levels presented in an image (256 in our case) for each distance d and orientation ϕ. The classification of texture is based on the characteristics extracted from the co-occurrence matrix: energy, entropy, maximum probability, contrast, inverse difference moment, and correlation. The three vectors of texture characteristics extracted from the three co-occurrence matrices are created using the six characteristics computed for $d = 1$ and $\phi = 0$. It results 18 values, used next in the content-based visual query.

The system offers the possibility to build the content-based visual query using color characteristic, texture characteristic, or a combination of them. The dissimilarity between images, taking into consideration color characteristic, is calculated using histograms intersection method, and for texture the Euclidian distance is used:

1. Euclidian distance for texture feature:

$$d_t = \sum_{m=0}^{M-1} (|h_q[m] - h_t[m]|)^2 \tag{2.1}$$

2. The intersection of the histograms for color feature [4]:

$$d_c = 1 - \frac{\sum_{m=0}^{M-1} \min(h_q[m], h_t[m]|)}{\min(h_q[m], h_t[m]|)} \tag{2.2}$$

If both distances are used in the query, the total distance is arithmetical average between the distances:

$$D = \frac{d_c + d_t}{2} \tag{2.3}$$

2.4 Evaluation of the Content-Based Image Retrieval Task

The experiments were performed on a database with 2,000 color medical images. For each query, the relevant images have been established. Each of the relevant images has become in its turn a query image, and the final results for a query are an average of these individual results. The values in Table 2.1 represent the number of relevant images (RLI) in the first 5/10 retrieved images, for some diagnoses.

In Fig. 2.1, there is an example of content-based image query considering the color and the texture feature. It can be observed a number of four relevant images in the first five retrieved and a number of six relevant images in the first ten retrieved (Fig. 2.2).

Many other experiments and comparative studies on medical images from digestive tract are presented in [20].

Table 2.1 The experimental results

Query	RLI/first five retrieved	RLI/first ten retrieved
Polyps	3	6
Colitis	4	7
Ulcer	3	6
Ulcerous tumor	3	5
Esophagitis	3	6

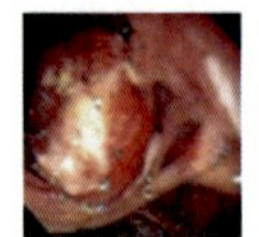

Fig. 2.1 Query image

Results					
Image					
Status	relevant	relevant	relevant	Irrelevant	relevant

Results					
Image					
Status	irrelevant	relevant	irrelevant	Irrelevant	relevant

Fig. 2.2 Content-based image retrieval—experimental results

2.5 Conclusions

As the values in the table and other experiments have shown, the content-based image retrieval applied on medical color images from the field of digestive apparatus finished with good results.

An important observation has to be done, which leads to the improvement of the quality of the content-based query on this type of images. For each query, at least in half of the cases, the color texture method based on co-occurrence matrices has given at least one relevant image for the query, image that could not be found using the color feature.

Both feature detection methods have the same complexity O(width*height), where width and height are the image dimensions. The two computed distances, the histogram intersection and the Euclidian distance, are equally complex O(m*n) where m is the number of values in the characteristics vector, and n is the number of images in the database.

The execution of the content-based image retrieval process also considering the color texture feature and the color feature leads to better results due to the fact that there are digestive track diagnostics which present not only color changes but also texture changes such as scratches and bruises.

References

1. Wong TCS (1998) Medical image databases. The springer international series in engineering and computer science, Springer, Dordrecht
2. Del Bimbo A (2001) Visual information retrieval. Morgan Kaufmann Publishers, San Francisco
3. Faloutsos C (2005) Searching multimedia databases by content. Springer, Dordrecht
4. Smith JR (1997) Integrated spatial and feature image systems: retrieval, compression and analysis. Ph.D. thesis, Graduate School of Arts and Sciences, Columbia University
5. Muller H, Michoux N, Bandon D, Geissbuhler A (2004) A review of content-based image retrieval systems in medical application – clinical benefits and future directions. Int J Med Inform 73(1):1–23
6. Muller H, Rosset A, Garcia A, Vallee JP, Geissbuhler A (2005) Benefits of content-based visual data access in radiology. Radio Graph 25:849–858
7. Gevers T (2004) Image search engines: an overview. Emerging topics in computer vision. Prentice Hall, Englewood Cliffs
8. Yong R, Thomas SH, Shih-Fu C (1999) Image retrieval: current techniques, promising directions, and open issues. J Vis Commun Image Representation 10:39–62
9. Flickner M, Sawhney H, Niblack W, Ashley J, Huang Q, Dom B, Gorkani M, Hafner J, Lee D, Petkovic D, Steele D, Yanker P (1999) Query by image and video content: the QBIC system. IEEE Comput 28(9):23–32
10. Qin H (1997) An evaluation on MARS – an image indexing and retrieval system. Graduate School of Library and Information Science, University of Illinois at Urbana-Champaign
11. Virginia EO, Stonebraker M (1995) Chabot: retrieval from a relational database of images. IEEE Comput 28(9):40–48
12. Smith JR, Chang SF (1996) Local color and texture extraction and spatial query. In: IEEE International conference on image processing, Lausanne, 1996
13. Smith JR, Chang SF (1996) Tools and techniques for color image retrieval. In: Symposium on electronic imaging: science and technology – storage & retrieval for image and video databases IV, San Jose, 1996, IS&T/SPIE, 2670
14. Smith JR, Chang SF (1997) SaFe: a general framework for integrated spatial and feature image search. In: IEEE signal processing society 1997 workshop on multimedia signal processing, Princetown, 1997
15. Carson C, Thomas M, Belongie S, Hellerstein JM, Malik J (1999) Blobworld: a system for region based image indexing and retrieval. In: Third international conference on visual information systems, lecture notes in computer science, vol 1614. Springer, Amsterdam, pp 509–516
16. IRMA Project (2007) http://phobos.imib.rwth-aachen.de/irma/index_en.php. Accessed 24.08.2011

17. Thies C, Güld MO, Fischer B, Lehmann TM (2005) Content-based queries on the CasImage database within the IRMA framework. A field report. LNCS 3491(59):781–792
18. Purdue University. Content-based Image Retrieval from Large Medical Image Databases. https://engineering.purdue.edu/RVL/Projects/CBIR/. Accessed 24.08.2011
19. Shyu C, Brodley CE, Kak AC, Kosaka A (1999) ASSERT: a physician-in-the-loop content-based retrieval system for HRCT image databases. Comput Vision Image Understanding 75:111–132
20. Stanescu L, Burdescu DD (2009) Multimedia medical databases. In: Sidhu AS, Dillon T, Bellgard M (eds) Biomedical data and applications, series: studies in computational intelligence, vol 224. Springer, Dordrecht

Chapter 3
Medical Images Segmentation

3.1 Introduction

The problem of partitioning images into homogenous regions or semantic entities is a basic problem for identifying relevant objects. There is a wide range of computational vision problems that could use of segmented images. For instance, intermediate-level vision problems motion estimation and tracking require determination of objects from frames. Higher-level problems such as object recognition and image indexing can also make use of segmentation results in matching, to address problems such as figure-ground separation and recognition by parts. In both intermediate-level and higher-level vision problems, contour detection of objects in real images is a fundamental problem. However, the problems of image segmentation and grouping remain nowadays a great challenge for computer vision. Visual saliency is related to some semantic concepts because certain parts of a scene are preattentively distinctive and have a greater significance than other parts. Objects are defined as visually distinguishable image compounds that can characterize visual properties of corresponding object classes, and they have been proposed as an effective middle-level representation of image content. An important approach for object detection is segmentation, and developing an accurate image segmentation technique which partitions image into salient regions is an important step. Unfortunately, the goal of the most part of the region detection techniques is to extract a single object in the image. Also, the ground truth for the most objects' databases indicates the single most salient structure in each image. However, many real images contain multiple salient structures, and the most salient structure may not be unambiguously defined. As a consequence, we consider that a segmentation method can detect visual objects from images if it can detect at least the most salient object. In this chapter, we study the segmentation problem in a general framework of image indexing and semantic image processing, where information extracted from detected visual objects, including color features of regions and geometric features of regions and contours, will be further used for image indexing and semantic processing. We have developed a region-based, computationally efficient,

L. Stanescu et al., *Creating New Medical Ontologies for Image Annotation: A Case Study*, SpringerBriefs in Electrical and Computer Engineering,
DOI 10.1007/978-1-4614-1909-9_3,

segmentation method that captures both certain perceptually important local and nonlocal image characteristics. In the following, our segmentation method will be denoted by graph-based object detection (GBOD).

Region-based segmentation methods can be broadly classified as either top-down (model-based) [1, 2] or bottom-up (visual feature-based) approaches [3, 4]. We have developed a visual feature-based method which uses a graph constructed on a hexagonal structure containing half of the image pixels in order to determine a forest of spanning trees for connected component representing visual objects. Thus, the image segmentation is treated as a graph partitioning problem. Many approaches aim to create large regions using simple homogeneity criteria based only on color or texture. However, applications for such approaches are limited as they often fail to create meaningful partitions due to either the complexity of the scene or difficult lighting conditions. We have determined the segmentation of a color image in two distinct steps: a presegmentation step, when only color information is used in order to determine an initial segmentation; and a syntactic-based segmentation step, when we define a predicate for determining the set of nodes of connected components based both on the color distance and geometric properties of regions. The novelty of our method concerns: (a) the virtual hexagonal structure used in the unified framework for image segmentation, (b) the using of maximum spanning trees for determining the set of nodes representing the connected components in the presegmentation step, (c) an adaptive method to determine the thresholds used both in the presegmentation and in the segmentation step, and (d) an automatic stopping criterion used in the segmentation step.

In addition our segmentation algorithm produces good results both from the perspective of perceptual grouping and from the perspective of determining relevant regions in the input images. We refer the term of perceptual grouping as a general expectation for a segmentation algorithm to produce perceptually coherent segmentation of regions at a level comparable to humans.

3.2 Related Work

Segmentation of medical images is the task of partitioning the data into contiguous regions representing individual anatomical objects. This task plays a vital role in many biomedical imaging applications: the quantification of tissue volumes, diagnosis, localization of pathology, study of anatomical structure, treatment planning, partial volume correction of functional imaging data, and computer-integrated surgery.

Segmentation is a difficult task because in most cases it is very hard to separate the object from the image background. Also, the image acquisition process brings noise in the medical data. Moreover, inhomogeneities in the data might lead to undesired boundaries. The medical experts can overcome these problems and identify objects in the data due to their knowledge about typical shape and image data characteristics. But manual segmentation is a very time-consuming process for the already increasing amount of medical images. As a result, reliable automatic methods for image segmentation are necessary.

It cannot be said that there is a segmentation method for medical images that produces good results for all types of images. There have been studied several segmentation methods that are influenced by factors like application domain, imaging modality, or others [5–7].

The segmentation methods were grouped in categories. Some of these categories are: thresholding, region growing, classifiers, clustering, Markov random field models, artificial neural networks, deformable models, or graph partitioning. Of course, there are other important methods that do not belong to any of these categories [6]. In thresholding approaches, an intensity value called the threshold must be established. This value will separate the image intensities in two classes: all pixels with intensity greater than the threshold are grouped into one class and all the other pixels into another class. If more than one threshold is determined, the process is called multithresholding.

Region growing is a technique for extracting a region from an image that contains pixels connected by some predefined criteria, based on intensity information and/or edges in the image. In its simplest form, region growing requires a seed point that is manually selected by an operator and extracts all pixels connected to the initial seed having the same intensity value. It can be used particularly for emphasizing small and simple structures such as tumors and lesions [6, 8].

Classifier methods represent pattern recognition techniques that try to partition a feature space extracted from the image using data with known labels. A feature space is the range space of any function of the image, with the most common feature space being the image intensities themselves. Classifiers are known as supervised methods because they need training data that are manually segmented by medical experts and then used as references for automatically segmenting new data [6, 7].

Clustering algorithms work as classifier methods, but they do not use training data. As a result, they are called unsupervised methods. Because there is not any training data, clustering methods iterate between segmenting the image and characterizing the properties of the each class. It can be said that clustering methods train themselves using the available data [6, 7, 9, 10].

Markov random field (MRF) is a statistical model that can be used within segmentation methods. For example, MRFs are often incorporated into clustering segmentation algorithms such as the K-means algorithm under a Bayesian prior model. MRFs model spatial interactions between neighboring or nearby pixels. In medical imaging, they are typically used to take into account the fact that most pixels belong to the same class as their neighboring pixels. In physical terms, this implies that any anatomical structure that consists of only one pixel has a very low probability of occurring under a MRF assumption [6, 7].

Artificial neural networks (ANNs) are massively parallel networks of processing elements or nodes that simulate biological learning. Each node in an ANN is capable of performing elementary computations. Learning is possible through the adaptation of weights assigned to the connections between nodes [6, 7]. ANNs are used in many ways for image segmentation.

Deformable models are physically motivated, model-based techniques for outlining region boundaries using closed parametric curves or surfaces that deform under the influence of internal and external forces. To outline an object boundary in an image, a closed curve or surface must be placed first near the desired boundary that comes into an iterative relaxation process [11–13].

To have an effective segmentation of images using varied image databases, the segmentation process has to be done based on the color and texture properties of the image regions [5, 14].

The automatic segmentation techniques were applied on various imaging modalities: brain imaging, liver images, chest radiography, computed tomography, digital mammography, or ultrasound imaging [6, 15, 16].

Finally, we briefly discuss the graph-based segmentation methods because they are most relevant to our work.

Most graph-based segmentation methods attempt to search certain structures in the associated edge-weighted graph constructed on the image pixels, such as minimum spanning tree [17, 18], or minimum cut [19, 20].

The major concept used in graph-based clustering algorithms is the concept of homogeneity of regions. For color segmentation algorithms, the homogeneity of regions is color-based, and thus the edge weights are based on color distance. Early graph-based methods [21] use fixed thresholds and local measures in finding segmentation. The segmentation criterion is to break the MST (minimum spanning trees) edges with the largest weight, which reflect the low-cost connection between two elements. To overcome the problem of fixed threshold, Urquhar [22] determined the normalized weight of an edge by using the smallest weight incident on the vertices touching that edge. Other methods [17, 18] use an adaptive criterion that depends on local properties rather than global ones. In contrast with the simple graph-based methods, cut-criterion methods capture the nonlocal properties of the image. The methods based on minimum cuts in a graph are designed to minimize the similarity between pixels that are being split [19, 20, 23]. The normalized cut criterion [19] takes into consideration self-similarity of regions. An alternative to the graph cut approach is to look for cycles in a graph embedded in the image plane. For example, in [24] the quality of each cycle is normalized in a way that is closely related to the normalized cuts approach.

Other approaches to image segmentation consist of splitting and merging regions according to how well each region fulfills some uniformity criterion. Such methods [25, 26] use a measure of uniformity of a region. In contrast, in [17, 18], a pairwise region comparison rather than applying a uniformity criterion to each individual region is used. Complex grouping phenomena can emerge from simple computation on these local cues [27].

A number of approaches to segmentation are based on finding compact clusters in some feature space [28, 29]. A recent technique using feature space clustering [30] first transforms the data by smoothing it in a way that preserves boundaries between regions. Color and motion have been studied in [31] with good results; however, these homogeneity criteria have some drawbacks for object extraction. Color cannot be used to characterize as a single region complex objects composed of several color-homogeneous parts. Another approach consists in extracting meaningful features from the available regions without restricting the analysis to specific objects. In [32], a new source of potentially important information to a wide range of segmentation applications which they term "syntactic features" is presented. Syntactic features represent geometric properties of regions and their spatial configurations. Examples of such features include homogeneity, compactness, regularity, inclusion, or symmetry.

The most part of approaches relating segmentation and relevant object determination use the notion of visual saliency. Usually, the visual saliency is defined as the perceptual quality that makes an object, person, or pixel stand out relative to its neighbors and thus capture human attention. The approaches for determining visual saliency can be based on biological models or purely computational ones. In general, all methods use some means of determining local contrast of image regions with their surroundings using one or more of the features of color, intensity, and orientation (see [33] for a recent survey). After the feature extraction, the second step consists on computation that is represented usually as a saliency map. Based on saliency maps, there are several approaches to perform the segmentation operation and thus to determine saliency objects from images. Achanta [34] uses a simple K-means algorithm based on the determined saliency map of an image for determining the salient regions of the image. Cao [35] uses an adaptive threshold to extract the region of interest (ROI) from the saliency map. Donoser [36] uses the region of interest extracted from the saliency map that is then used as an initialization step for the subsequent figure/ground segmentation. A different approach is given in [37] where some local, regional, and global features that define a salient object are introduced such as multiscale contrast, center-surround histogram, and color spatial distribution. The salient object detection problem is treated as a binary labeling problem by separating the salient object from the background, and the conditional random field (CRF) framework is used to learn an optimal linear combination of features. A common weakness of those approaches is the fact that they are computationally expensive, both for determining the saliency map and for learning the linear combination of features.

3.3 Graph-Based Image Segmentation Algorithm

Our previous work [38–41] is related to the works in [17, 18] in the sense of pairwise comparison of region similarity. We use different measures for internal contrast of a connected component and for external contrast between two connected components than the measures used in [17, 18].

The internal contrast of a component C represents the maximum weight of edges connecting vertices from C, and the external contrast between two components represents the maximum weight of edges connecting vertices from these two components. These measures are in our opinion closer to the human perception. We use maximum spanning tree instead of minimum spanning tree in the presegmentation

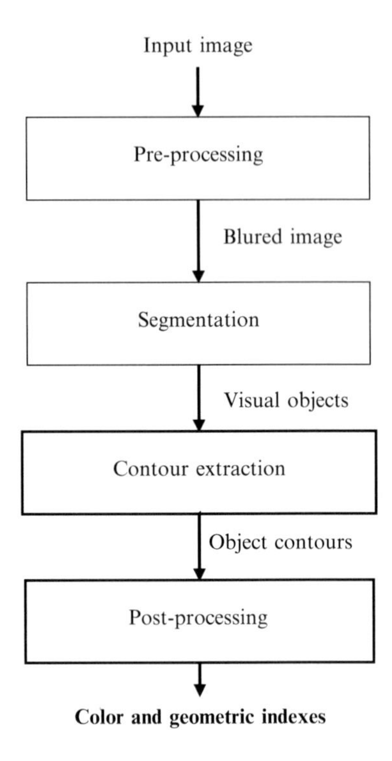

Fig. 3.1 Structure of the image processing system

step in order to manage external contrast between connected components. Concerning the final segmentation step, we use the notion of syntactic attributes of regions as defined in [32, 42] together with color features of regions in order to determine dynamic weights of edges and the order to merge adjacent edges. We use in this case minimum spanning trees and a graph contraction procedure in order to determine salient regions from images.

The low-level system for image segmentation and boundary extraction of visual objects described in this section is designed to be integrated in a general framework of indexing and semantic image processing. The framework uses color and geometric features of image regions in order to (a) determine relevant visual objects and their contours and also (b) to extract specific color and geometric information from these objects to be further used into a higher-level image processing system.

The proposed multilevel image processing system is presented in Fig. 3.1, and it contains four modules that can be integrated into a semantic image processing system for shape representation and retrieval. The preprocessing module is used mainly to blur the initial RGB image in order to reduce the image noise by applying a 2D Gaussian kernel [43].

The segmentation module creates a virtual hexagonal structure on the pixels of the input image and a triangular grid graph having hexagons as vertices. In order to allow a unitary processing for the multilevel system at this level, we store, for each determined component C, the set of the hexagons contained in the region associated to C and the set of hexagons located at the boundary of the component. In addition, for each component, the dominant color of the region is extracted. This color will be further used in the postprocessing module. The contour extraction module determines for each segment of the image its boundary. The boundaries of the determined visual objects are closed contours represented by a sequence of adjacent hexagons. At this level, a linked list of points representing the contour is added to each determined component. The postprocessing module extracts representative information for the above determined visual objects and their contours in order to create an efficient index for a semantic image processing system.

An image processing task contains mainly three important components: acquisition, processing, and visualization. After the acquisition stage, an image is sampled at each point on a two-dimensional grid storing intensity or color information and implicit location information for each sample. The rectangular grid is the most dominant of any grid structure in image processing, and conventional acquisition devices acquire square-sampled images. The processing stage uses in this case a square lattice model of the input image. An important advantage of using rectangular grid is the fact that the visualization stage uses directly the square pixels of the digitized image. Another two-dimensional grid used in the image processing stages is the hexagonal grid [44–46]. The hexagonal structured pixel grid is considered to be superior to the rectangular grid system in many respects, including greater angular resolution, and the consistent connectivity [44, 45]. The algorithms of the processing stage use in this case a hexagonal lattice model of the input image [45]. Because conventional acquisition devices acquire square-sampled images, a common approach to acquiring hexagonally sampled images is to convert the input image from a square lattice to a hexagonal lattice, a process known as image resampling.

We do not use a hexagonal lattice model because of the additional actions involving the double conversion between square and hexagonal pixels. However, we intent to use some of the advantages of the hexagonal grid such as uniform connectivity. In this case, only one type of neighborhood is possible in the hexagonal grid, the 6-neighborhood structure, unlike several types as N4 and N8 in the case of square lattice. This implies that there will be less ambiguity in defining boundaries and regions [45]. As a consequence, we construct a virtual hexagonal structure over the square pixels of an input image, as presented in Fig. 3.2. This virtual hexagonal grid is not a hexagonal lattice because the constructed hexagons are not regular.

Let I be an initial image having the dimension $w \times h$ (e.g., a matrix having h rows and w columns of square pixels). In order to construct a hexagonal grid on these pixels, we retain an eventually smaller image with:

$$h' = h - (h - 1) \bmod 2 \quad \text{and} \quad w' = w - (w \bmod 2) \tag{3.1}$$

In the reduced image, at most the last line of pixels and at most the last three columns of pixels are lost, assuming that for the initial image $h > 3$ and $w > 4$, that is, a convenient restriction for input images. Each hexagon from the hexagonal grid

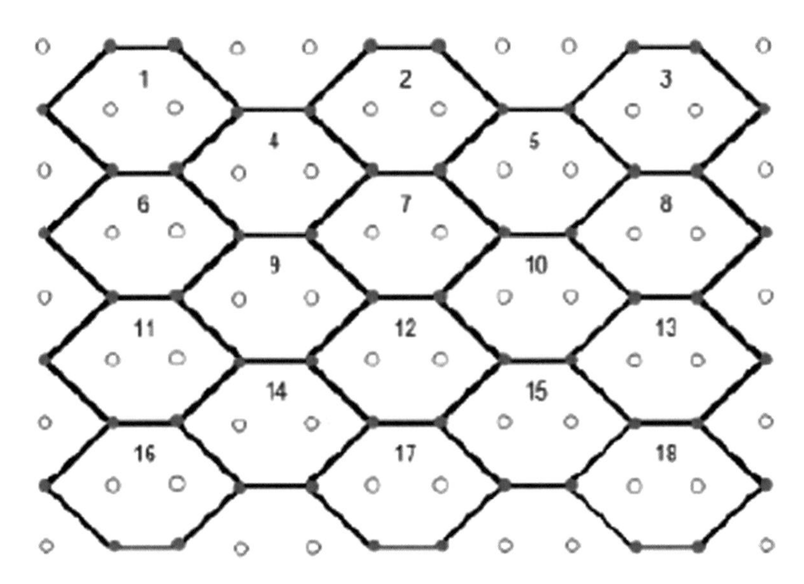

Fig. 3.2 Hexagonal structure constructed on the image pixels

contains eight pixels: six pixels from the frontier and two interior pixels. Because square pixels from an image have integer values as coordinates, we select always the left pixel from the two interior pixels to represent with approximation the gravity center of the hexagon, denoted by the pseudogravity center. We use a simple scheme of addressing for the hexagons of the hexagonal grid that encodes the spatial location of the pseudogravity centers of the hexagons as presented in Fig. 3.2.

Let $w \times h$ the dimension of the initial image verifying the previous restriction (e.g., $h \bmod 2 = 1$, $w \bmod 4 = 0$, $h \geq 3$, and $w \geq 4$). Given the coordinates $< h, c >$ of a pixel "p" from the input image, we use the linearized function, $ip_{w,h}(h,c) = (1 - 1)w + c$, in order to determine an unique index for the pixel.

Let "ps" be the subsequence of the pixels from the sequence of the pixels of the initial image that correspond to the pseudogravity center of hexagons and "hs" the sequence of hexagons constructed over the pixels of the initial image. For each pixel p from the sequence "ps" having the coordinates $< h, c>$, the index of the corresponding hexagon from the sequence "hs" is given by the following relation:

$$fh_{w,h}(h,c) = [(l-2)w + c - 2l]/4 + 1 \tag{3.2}$$

It is easy to verify the following two properties related to the function *fh*:

1. The value $[(l - 2)w + c - 2l]$ is always divisible by 4.
2. Let "p" be a pixel from the subsequence "ps" of pixels representing the pseudogravity center of hexagons, having the coordinates $<h,c>$, and i its index in this subsequence, $p = ps_i$. In this case, the following relation holds:

$$fh_{w,h}(h,c) = i \tag{3.3}$$

This remark states in fact that the scheme of addressing for the hexagons is linear, and it has a natural order induced by the subsequence of pixels representing the pseudogravity center of hexagons.

Moreover, it is easy to verify that the function *fh* defined by the relation (3.2) is bijective. Its inverse function is given by:

$$fh^{-1}{}_{w,h}(k) = \langle 1, c \rangle \tag{3.4}$$

where

$$l = \begin{cases} 2 + [4(k-1)]/w, & \text{if} : h < w \\ 2 + [4(k-1)]/w + tw, & \text{if} : h \geq w, \quad \text{and} : h = tw + h' \end{cases} \tag{3.5}$$

$$c = 4(k-1) + 2l - (l-2)w \tag{3.6}$$

Relations (3.4), (3.5), and (3.6) allow to uniquely determining the coordinates of the pixel representing the pseudogravity center of a hexagon specified by its index (its address). In addition, these relations allow us to determine the sequence of coordinates of all eight pixels contained into a hexagon with an address k:

$$\begin{aligned} \mathrm{p8}(k) = \langle & \langle l-1, c\rangle, \langle l-1, c+1\rangle, \langle l, c+2\rangle, \langle l+1, c+1\rangle, \\ & \langle l+1, c\rangle, \langle l, c-1\rangle, \langle l, c\rangle, \langle l, c+1\rangle \rangle \end{aligned} \tag{3.7}$$

where $\langle l, c \rangle = fh^{-1}{}_{w,h}(k)$ from (3.4)

The subsequence "ps" of the pixels representing the pseudogravity center and the function *fh* defined by the relation (3.2) allow to determine the sequence of the hexagons "hs" that is used by the segmentation and contour detection algorithms.

After the processing step, the relations (3.4), (3.5), (3.6), and (3.7) allow to update the pixels of the initial image for the visualization step. Each hexagon represents an elementary item, and the entire virtual hexagonal structure represents a triangular grid graph, $G = (V,E)$, where each hexagon h in this structure has a corresponding vertex vV. The set E of edges is constructed by connecting hexagons that are neighbors in a 6-connected sense. The vertices of this graph correspond to the pseudogravity centers of the hexagons from the hexagonal grid, and the edges are straight lines connecting the pseudogravity centers of the neighboring hexagons, as presented in Fig. 3.3.

There are two main advantages when using hexagons instead of pixels as elementary piece of information:

1. The amount of memory space associated to the graph vertices is reduced. Denoting by "np" the number of pixels of the initial image, the number of the resulted hexagons is always less than np/4, and thus the cardinal of both sets V and E is significantly reduced.

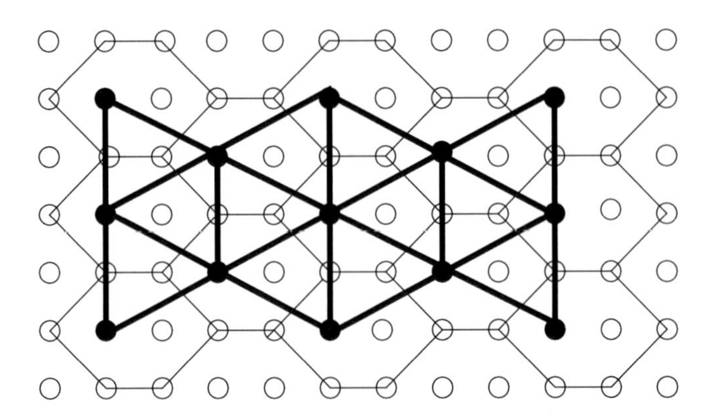

Fig. 3.3 The triangular grid graph constructed on the pseudogravity centers of the hexagonal grid

2. The algorithms for determining the visual objects and their contours are much faster and simpler in this case.

We associate to each hexagon h from V two important attributes representing its dominant color and the coordinates of its pseudogravity center, denoted by $g(h)$. The dominant color of a hexagon is denoted by $c(h)$, and it represents the color of the pixel of the hexagon which has the minimum sum of color distance to the other seven pixels. Each hexagon h in the hexagonal grid is thus represented by a single point, $g(h)$, having the color $c(h)$. By using the values $g(h)$ and $c(h)$ for each hexagon, information related to all pixels from the initial image is taken into consideration by the segmentation algorithm.

Let $V = \{h_1, \ldots, h_{|V|}\}$ be the set of hexagons constructed on the image pixels as presented previously and $G = (V,E)$ be the undirected grid graph, with E containing pairs of hexagons that are neighbors in a 6-connected sense. The weight of each edge $e = (h_i,h_j)$ is denoted by $w(e)$, or similarly by $w(h_i,h_j)$, and it represents the dissimilarity between neighboring elements h_i and h_j in some feature space. Components of an image represent compact regions containing pixels with similar properties. Thus, the set V of vertices of the graph G is partitioned into disjoint sets, each subset representing a distinct visual object of the initial image.

As in other graph-based approaches [17], we use the notion of segmentation of the set V. A segmentation, S, of V is a partition of V such that each component $C \in S$ corresponds to a connected component in a spanning subgraph $G_S = (V, E_S)$ of G, with $E_S \subseteq E$.

The set of edges $E - E_S$ that are eliminated connects vertices from distinct components. The common boundary between two connected components $C', C'' \in S$ represents the set of edges connecting vertices from the two components:

$$cb(C',C'') = \{(h_i, h_j) \in E | h_i \in C', h_j \in C''\} \tag{3.8}$$

The set of edges $E - E_S$ represents the boundary between all components in S. This set is denoted by *bound*(S), and it is defined as follows:

$$bound(S) = \bigcup_{C', C'' \in S} cb(C', C'') \tag{3.9}$$

In order to simplify notations throughout the paper, we use C_i to denote the component of a segmentation S that contains the vertex $h_i \in E$.

We use the notions of segmentation too fine and too coarse as defined in [17] that attempt to formalize the human perception of relevant visual objects from an image. A segmentation S is too fine if there is some pair of components $C', C'' \in S$ for which there is no evidence for a boundary between them. A segmentation S is too coarse when there exists a proper refinement of S that is not too fine. The key element in this definition is the evidence for a boundary between two components.

The goal of a segmentation method is to determine a proper segmentation, which represent relevant objects from an image.

Definition 1

Let $G = (V,E)$ be the undirected graph constructed on the hexagonal structure of an image, with $V = \{h_1, \ldots, h_{|V|}\}$. A proper segmentation of V is a partition S of V such that there exists a sequence $<S^i, S^{i+1}, \ldots, S^{f-1}, S^f>$ of segmentations of V for which:

1. $S = S^f$ is the final segmentation, and S^i is the initial segmentation.
2. S^j is a proper refinement of S^{j+1} (i.e., $S^j \subset S^{j+1}$) for each $j = i, \ldots, f - 1$.
3. Segmentation S^j is too fine, for each $j = i, \ldots, f - 1$.
4. Any segmentation S^l such that $S^f \subset S^l$ is too coarse.
5. Segmentation S^f is neither too coarse nor too fine.

In the above definition, S^a is a refinement of S^b in the sense of partitions, that is, every set in S^a is a subset of one of the sets in S^b. We say that S^a is a proper refinement of S^b if S^a is a refinement of S^b and $S^a \neq S^b$. In the case of a proper refinement, S^a is obtained by splitting one or more components from S^b, or similarly, S^b is obtained by merging one or more components from S^a. Let $C', C'' \in S^a$ be two components obtained by splitting a component $C \in S^b$. In this case, C' and C'' have a common boundary, $cb(C', C'') \neq \Phi$..

Our segmentation algorithm starts with the most refined segmentation, $S^0 = \{\{h_1\}, \ldots, \{h_{|V|}\}\}$, and it constructs a sequence of segmentations until a proper segmentation is achieved. Each segmentation S^j is obtained from the segmentation.

S^{j-1} by merging two or more connected components, for there is no evidence for a boundary between them. For each component of a segmentation, a spanning tree is constructed, and thus for each segmentation, we use an associated spanning forest.

The evidence for a boundary between two components is determined taking into consideration some features in some model of the image. When starting, for a certain number of segmentations, the only considered feature is the color of the regions associated to the components, and in this case we use a color-based region model.

When the components became complex and contain too much hexagons, the color model is not sufficient, and geometric features together with color information are considered. In this case, we use a syntactic based with a color-based region model for regions. In addition, syntactic features bring supplementary information for merging similar regions in order to determine relevant objects. For the sake of simplicity, we will denote this region model as syntactic-based region model.

As a consequence, we split the sequence of all segmentations,

$$S_{if} = \langle S^0, S^1, \ldots, S^{k-1}, S^k \rangle \tag{3.10}$$

in two different subsequences, each subsequence having a different region model,

$$\begin{aligned} S_i &= \langle S^0, S^1, \ldots, S^{t-1}, S^t \rangle \\ S_f &= \langle S^t, S^{t+1}, \ldots, S^{k-1}, S^k \rangle \end{aligned} \tag{3.11}$$

where S_i represents the color-based segmentation sequence, and S_f represents the syntactic-based segmentation sequence. The final segmentation S^t in the color-based model is also the initial segmentation in the syntactic-based region model.

For each sequence of segmentations, we develop a different algorithm. Moreover, we use a different type of spanning tree in each case: a maximum spanning tree in the case of the color-based segmentation and a minimum spanning tree in the case of the syntactic-based segmentation. More precisely, our method determines two sequences of forests of spanning trees,

$$\begin{aligned} F^i &= \langle F_0, F_1, \ldots, F_{t-1}, F_t \rangle \\ F^f &= \langle F'_t, F'_{t+1}, \ldots, F'_{k-1}, F'_k \rangle \end{aligned} \tag{3.12}$$

each sequence of forests being associated to a sequence of segmentations.

The first forest from F^i contains only the vertices of the initial graph, $F_0 = (V, \Phi)$, and at each step, some edges from E are added to the forest $F_l = (V, E^l)$ to obtain the next forest, $F_{l+1} = (V, E^{l+1})$. The forests from F^i contain maximum spanning trees, and they are determined by using a modified version of Kruskal's algorithm, where at each step, the heaviest edge (u,v) that leaves the tree associated to u is added to the set of edges of the current forest.

The second subsequence of forests that correspond to the subsequence of segmentations S_f contains forests of minimum spanning trees, and they are determined by using a modified form of Boruvka's algorithm. This sequence uses as input a new graph, $G' = (V',E')$, which is extracted from the last forest, F_t, of the sequence F^i. Each vertex v from the set V' corresponds to a component Cv from the segmentation S^t (i.e., to a region determined by the previous algorithm).

At each step, the set of new edges added to the current forest is determined by each tree T contained in the forest that locates the lightest edge leaving T. The first forest from F^f contains only the vertices of the graph $G', F't = (V', \Phi)$.

There are many existing systems for arranging and describing colors, such as RGH, YUV, HSV, LUV, CIELAV, Munsell system, etc. [47]. We have decided to use the RGB color space because it is efficient, and no conversion is required. Although it also suffers from the nonuniformity problem where the same distance between two color points within the color space may be perceptually quite different in different parts of the space, within a certain color threshold, it is still definable in terms of color consistency.

In the color model, regions are modeled by a vector in the RGB color space. This vector is the mean color value of the dominant color of hexagons belonging to the regions.

The evidence for a boundary between two regions is based on the difference between the internal contrast of the regions and the external contrast between them [17]. Both notions of internal contrast and external contrast between two regions are based on the dissimilarity between two colors.

We have chosen the definition of the external contrast between two components to be the maximum weight edge connecting the two components and not to be the minimum weight as in [17] because: (a) it is closer to the human perception (in the sense of the perception of the maximum color dissimilarity), and (b) the contrast is uniformly defined (as maximum color dissimilarity) in the two cases of internal and external contrast.

Let $G = (V,E)$ be the initial graph constructed on the hexagonal structure of an image. The proposed segmentation algorithm will produce a proper segmentation of V according to the definition 1. The sequence of segmentations, S_{if}, as defined by Eq. 3.10, and its associated sequence of forests of spanning trees, F^{if}, as defined by Eq. 3.12, will be iteratively generated as follows:

1. The color-based sequence of segmentations, S_i, as defined by Eq. 3.11, and its associated sequence of forests, F^i, as defined by Eq. 3.12, will be generated by using the color-based region model and a maximum spanning tree construction method based on a modified form of the Kruskal's algorithm.
2. The syntactic-based sequence of segmentations, S_f, as defined by Eq. 3.11, and its associated sequence of forests, F^f, as defined by Eq. 3.12, will be generated by using the syntactic-based model and a minimum spanning tree construction method based on a modified form of the Boruvka's algorithm.

The general form of the segmentation procedure is presented in algorithm 1

Algorithm 1: Segmentation algorithm

1: **Procedure** SEGMENTATION(*l*, *c*, *P*, *H*, *Comp*)
2: **Input** *l*, *c*, *P*
3: **Output** *H*, *Comp*
4: $H \leftarrow$CREATEHEXAGONALSTRUCTURE(*l*, *c*, *P*)
5: $G \leftarrow$CREATEINITIALGRAPH(*l*, *c*, *P*, *H*)
6: CREATECOLORPARTITION(*G*, *H*, *Bound*)
7: $G' \leftarrow$EXTRACTGRAPH(*G*, *Bound*, th^k_g)
8: CREATESYNTACTICPARTITION(*G*, *G'*, th^k_g)
9: $Comp \leftarrow$EXTRACTFINALCOMPONENTS(*G'*)
10: **End procedure**

The input parameters represent the image resulted after the preprocessing operation: the array *P* of the image pixels structured in "*l*" lines and "*c*" columns. The output parameters of the segmentation procedure will be used by the contour extraction procedure: the hexagonal grid stored in the array of hexagons *H* and the array Comp representing the set of determined components associated to the salient objects in the input image.

The color-based segmentation and the syntactic-based segmentation are determined by the procedures CREATECOLORPARTITION and CREATESYNTACTICPARTITION respectively.

The color-based and syntactic-based segmentation algorithms use the hexagonal structure *H* created by the function CREATEHEXAGONALSTRUCTURE over the pixels of the initial image and the initial triangular grid graph *G* created by the function CREATEINITIALGRAPH. Because the syntactic-based segmentation algorithm uses a graph contraction procedure, CREATESYNTACTICPARTITION uses a different graph, G', extracted by the procedure EXTRACTGRAPH after the color-based segmentation finishes.

Both algorithms for determining the color-based and syntactic-based segmentation use and modify a global variable (denoted by *CC*) with two important roles:

1. To store relevant information concerning the growing forest of spanning trees during the segmentation (maximum spanning trees in the case of the color-based segmentation and minimum spanning trees in the case of syntactic-based segmentation)
2. To store relevant information associated to components in a segmentation in order to extract the final components because each tree in the forest represents in fact a component in each segmentation *S* in the segmentation sequence determined by the algorithm

In addition, this variable is used to maintain a fast disjoint set structure in order to reduce the running time of the color-based segmentation algorithm. The variable *CC* is an array having the same dimension as the array of hexagons *H*, which contains as elements objects of the class Tree with the following associated fields:

(isRoot, parent, compIndex, frontier, surface, color)

The field "isRoot" is a Boolean value specifying if the corresponding hexagon index is the root of a tree representing a component, and the field parent represents the index of the hexagon which is the parent of the current hexagon. The rest of the fields are used only if the field "isRoot" is true. The field "compIndex" is the index of the associated component.

The field "surface" is a list of indices of the hexagons belonging to the associated component, while the field "frontier" is a list of indices of the hexagons belonging to the frontier of the associated component. The field color is the mean color of the hexagon colors of the associated component.

The procedure EXTRACTFINALCOMPONENTS determines for each determined component *C* of Comp, the set *sa*(*C*) of hexagons belonging to the component, the set $sp(C)$ of hexagons belonging to the frontier, and the dominant color $c(C)$ of the component.

Let $G = (V,E)$ be the undirected graph constructed on the hexagonal structure of an image. The color-based segmentation algorithm will produce a proper segmentation of V according to the definition 1. The sequence of segmentations, $<S^0, S^1,\ldots,S^{t-1}, S^t>$, and its associated sequence of growing forests, $<F_0, F_1,\ldots, F_{t-1}, F_t>$, will be iteratively generated, based on a maximum spanning tree construction method. We use a modified form of the Kruskal's algorithm presented in algorithm 2, where the trees generated at each step represent the connected components of segmentation.

Algorithm 2: Color-based segmentation

```
 1: Procedure CREATECOLORPARTITION(G, H, Bound)
 2: Input G = (V,E), H = {h1, . . .,h|V|}
 3: Output Bound
 4: t←DETERMINETHRESHOLD(G)
 5: Bound ←hi ◁Initialize Bound
 6: for all i←1, |V| do
 7: MAKESET(hi) ◁Initialize the disjoint set data structures
 8: end for
 9:     ◁ At this point l ←0
10:     ◁ and S0 ←{{h1}, . . . ,{h|V|}}
11: SORT(E,Ep)
12:     ◁ Ep = he p1 , . . ., e p|E| i is the sorting of E
13:       ◁ in order of non-increasing weight
14: for all k←1, |E| do
15:     ◁ Let e pk = (hi ,hj) be the current edge in Ep
16: ti ←FINDSET(hi)
17: t j ←FINDSET(hj)
18: if ti 6=t j then
19: if w(hi ,hj) ≤ INTVAR(ti, t j)+ t(ti, t j) then
20: UNION(ti, t j,w(hi,hj))
21:     ◁ l ←l+1
22:       ◁ Sl ←Sl−1−{{Cti},{Ct j }}S{Cti ∪ Ct j }
23: else
24: Add the edge (hi ,hj) the the list Bound
25: ◁ bound(Sl )←bound(Sl−1)∪ {(hi,hj)}
26: end if
27: else
28:     ◁Do nothing, ti ∈ Ct j
29: end if
30: end for
31: End procedure
```

The input parameters of the color-based segmentation algorithm are the initial graph G and the array H of the hexagons from the hexagonal grid. The output parameter is the list "bound" of edges representing the boundary of the final segmentation.

Because we use maximum spanning trees instead of minimum spanning trees, the list of the edges $E(G)$ is sorted in nonincreasing edge weight. The forest of spanning trees is initialized in such a way each element of the forest contains exactly one hexagon.

For each segmentation S^1 determined by algorithm 2 and for each connected component C of the corresponding spanning graph G_1, there is a unique maximum spanning tree, $F_1(C)$, that maximizes the sum of edge weights for this component.

The forest of all maximum spanning trees associated to the segmentation S^1 is

$$F_1 = \bigcup_{c \in S_1} F_1(C) \tag{3.13}$$

and algorithm makes greedy decisions about which edges to add to F_1. Every time when an edge is added to the maximum spanning tree, a union of the two partial spanning trees containing the two vertices of the edge is made. In this way, the sequence of the edges contained in the forest F_1 of spanning trees is implicitly determined at the line 14 of algorithm 2. Conversely, for each tree T from the forest F_1, the set of all vertices of the initial graph contained in the tree T is denoted by $Set(T)$, and it represents the connected component of S^1 associated to maximum spanning tree T:

$$T = F_1(Set(T)) \tag{3.14}$$

The functions MAKESET, FINDSET, and UNION used by the segmentation algorithm implement the classical MAKESET, FIND-SET, and UNION operations for disjoint set data structures with union by rank and path compression [48]. In addition, the function call, UNION(t_i, t_j,$w(h_i,h_j)$), performs the following operation, assuming that t_i is the root of the new spanning tree resulted by combining the spanning trees represented by t_i and t_j:

1. Determining $CC[t_i]$.surface as the concatenation of the lists $CC[t_i]$.surface and $C[t_j]$.surface
2. Determining $CC[t_i]$.frontier as a list of indices of hexagons belonging to the frontier of the new component $\{Ct_i \cup Ct_j\}$
3. Determining $CC[t_i]$.color as the value $(n_i c_i + n_j c_j)/(n_i + n_j)$, where $c_i = CC[t_i]$.color, and n_i represents the number of elements in the tree $CC[t_i]$

In order to determine a good final segmentation and to discover the relevant objects from the input image, the syntactic-based sequence of segmentations, S_f, as defined by Eq. 3.11, can decomposed into several subsequences, each subsequence being determined by a modified form of the Boruvka's algorithm.

Let $i_1 < i_2 < \ldots < i_x < i_{x+1}$ be a sequence of indices, with $i_1 = t$ and $i_{x+1} = k$, that allows a decomposition of the sequence S_f as follows:

$$S_f = <S_{i1}, S_{i1+1}, \ldots, S_{i2-1}, S_{i2}, S_{i2+1}, S_{i2+2}, \ldots, S_{i3}, \ldots, S_{ix+1}, S_{ix+2}, \ldots S_{ix+1}> \tag{3.15}$$

As presented in algorithm 3, the procedure CREATESYNTACTICPARTITION implements the syntactic-based segmentation, while the function GENERATE-PARTITION is used to generate the subsequences of segmentations, $S_{f1}, \ldots, S_{fx}$, each subsequence of the form,

$$S_{fj} = <S^{ij}, S^{ij+1}, \ldots, S^{ij+1-1}, S^{ij+1}> \tag{3.16}$$

being determined by the function GENERATEPARTITION at the j-th call. The last segmentation of the subsequence S_{fj} generated by GENERATEPARTITION is also the input sequence of the (j +1)-th call of GENERATEPARTITION. The first input segmentation S^{i1} is the final segmentation S^t of the color-based segmentation algorithm. The function DETERMINEWEIGHTS determines the set A of weights.

Algorithm 3: Syntactic-based segmentation

1: **Procedure** CREATESYNTACTICPARTITION(G,G', th^k_g)
2: **Input** G, G', th^k_g
3: **Output** G'
4: A←DETERMINEWEIGHTS(G')
5: *count* ←0
6: **repeat**
7: G' ← GENERATEPARTITION(G,G', th^k_g,*newPart*)
8: **if** *newPart* **then**
9: *count* ←0
10: k←[a0 a0 a0 a0]T
11: **end if**
12: th^k_g ←MODIFYWEIGHTS(G', k)
13: *count* ←*count* +1
14: NEXTKVECTOR(k)
15: **until** *count* = |A|4
16: **End procedure**

More formally, the jth call of the function GENERATEPARTITION, for which the output parameter "newPart" has the value "true," is associated to the nonempty subsequence S_{fj} of segmentations, and it generates a sequence of graphs

$$G^{ij} = <G^{ij}_{ij}, G^{ij}_{ij+1}, \ldots, G^{ij}_{ij+1-1}, G^{ij}_{ij+1}> \tag{3.17}$$

and a sequence of associated forests of minimum spanning trees,

$$F^{ij} = <F^{ij}_{ij}, F^{ij}_{ij+1}, \ldots, F^{ij}_{ij+1-1}, F^{ij}_{ij+1}> \quad (3.18)$$

such that the last forest is empty, $\underline{F}^{ij}_{ij+1} = \Phi$. For each graph $G_1{}^{ij}$ from the sequence $\underline{G}^{ij}$, and $\underline{F}_1{}^{ij}$ represents the forest of minimum spanning trees of G^{ij}_1, and G^{ij}_{1+1} is the contraction of G^{ij}_1 over all the edges that appear in $\underline{F}_1{}^{ij}$.

Because the last graph, G^{ij}_{ij+1} of the sequence $\underline{G}^{ij}$ cannot be further contracted, the dissimilarity vectors of functions associated to the edge weights, $d(C(v_i),C(v_j))$, are not modified, and thus the edge weights, $w(v_i,v_j)$, are not modified. In order to restart the process for determining the new subsequence,

$$S_{f,j+1} = <S^{ij+1}, S^{ij+1+1}, \ldots, S^{ij+2}> \quad (3.19)$$

the first graph, G^{ij+1}_{ij+1} of the sequence $\underline{G}^{ij+1}$ differs from the last graph, G^{ij+1}_{ij+1} of the sequence $\underline{G}^{ij}$ by modifying only the weighted vector $k \in K$.

The function MODIFYWEIGHTS of algorithm 3 realizes this modification and recalculates the new global weighted threshold. In this case, the values for the weighted vector "*k*" are sequential determined in the lexicographic order, generated by the procedure NEXTKVECTOR.

This constraint is necessary in order to realize a stopping criterion for the algorithm: the last graph cannot be modified, and for all distinct values of the weighted vectors k $\in K$, and thus another partition cannot be determined.

Each time when GENERATEPARTITION generates a nonempty sequence of segmentations, the output parameter "newPart" became "true," and the first vector of the set K is generated. When GENERATEPARTITION generates an empty sequence of segmentations, "newPart" is false, and the next vector in lexicographic order is generated by the procedure NEXTKVECTOR.

When sequentially for all distinct weighted vectors $k \in K$ generated in lexicographic order the function GENERATEPARTITION generates an empty sequence of segmentations, the procedure CREATESYNTACTICPARTITION finishes. The function GENERATEPARTITION is a generalized greedy algorithm for constructing minimum spanning trees.

3.4 The Color Set Back-Projection Algorithm

Color sets provide an alternative to color histograms for representing color information. Their utilization is based on the assumption that salient regions have not more than few equally prominent colors.

The color set back-projection algorithm proposed in [49] is a technique for the automated extraction of regions and representation of their color content.

The back-projection process requires several stages: color set selection, back-projection onto the image, thresholding, and labeling. Candidate color sets are selected first with one color, then with two colors, etc., until the salient regions are extracted. For each, image is performed with a quantization of the RGB color space at 64 colors.

The algorithm follows the reduction of insignificant color information and makes evident the significant color regions, followed by the generation, in automatic way, of the regions of a single color, of the two colors, etc.

For each detected region, the color set, the area, and the localization are stored. The region localization is given by the minimal bounding rectangle. The region area is represented by the number of color pixels and can be smaller than the minimum bounding rectangle.

The image processing algorithm computes both the global histogram of the image and the binary color set. The quantized colors from 0 to 63 are stored in a matrix. To this matrix, a 5 × 5 median filter, which has the role of eliminating the isolated points, is applied. The process of regions' extraction is using the filtered matrix, and it is a depth—first traversal described in pseudocod in the following way:

```
Procedure FindRegions (Image I, colorset C)
 1)  InitStack(S)
 2)  Visited = ∅
 3)  for *each node P in the I do
 4)   if *color of P is in C then
 5)     PUSH(P)
 6)     Visited ← Visited ∪ {P}
 7)     while not Empty(S) do
 8)       CrtPoint ←POP()
 9)       Visited ← Visited ∪ {CrtPoint}
10)      For *each unvisited neighbor S of CrtPoint do
11)       if *color of S is in C then
12)         Visited ← Visited ∪ {S}
13)         PUSH(S)
14)       end
15)      end
16)  end
17) * Output detected region
18) end
19) end
```

The total running time for a call of the procedure FindRegions (Image I, colorset C) is $O(m^2 \times n^2)$ where m is the width and n is the height of the image [7].

3.5 The Local Variation Algorithm

This algorithm described in [17] is using a graph-based approach for the image segmentation process. The pixels are considered the graph nodes, so in this way it is possible to define an undirected graph $G = (V, E)$ where the vertices from V represent the set of elements to be segmented. Each edge (v_i,v_j) belonging to E has associated a corresponding weight $w(v_i,v_j)$ calculated based on color, which is a measure of the dissimilarity between neighboring elements v_i and v_j.

A minimum spanning tree is obtained using Kruskal's algorithm. The connected components that are obtained represent image's regions. It is supposed that the graph has m edges and n vertices. This algorithm is described also in [50] where it has four major steps that are presented below:

1. Sort $E = (e_1, \ldots, e_m)$ such that $|e_t| < -e_{t'}| \forall t < t'$.
2. Let $S^0 = (\{x_1, \ldots, \{x_n\})$ be each initial cluster containing only one vertex.
3. For $t = 1, \ldots, m$.
   (a) Let x_i and x_j be the vertices connected by e_t.
   (b) Let C_{xi}^{t-} be the connected component containing point x_i on iteration $t - 1$ and $l_i = \max_{mst} C^{t\ -\ 1}{}_{xi}$.
   Be the longest edge in the minimum spanning tree of C_{xi}^{t-1}. Likewise for l_j.
   (c) Merge C_{xi}^{t-1} and C_{xj}^{t-1} if $|e_t| < \min\{l_i + \frac{k}{C_{xi}^{t-1}}, l_j + \frac{k}{C_{xj}^{t-1}}\}$ where k is a constant.
4. $S = S^m$.

The existence of a boundary between two components in segmentation is based on a predicate D. This predicate is measuring the dissimilarity between elements along the boundary of the two components relative to a measure of the dissimilarity among neighboring elements within each of the two components. The internal difference of a component $C \subseteq V$ was defined as the largest weight in the minimum spanning tree of a component MST(C, E):

$$Int(C) = \max_{e \in MST(CE)} w(e) \tag{3.20}$$

The difference between two components $C_1, C_2 \subset V$ is defined as the minimum weight edge connecting the two components:

$$Dif(C_1, C_2) = \min_{v_i \in C_1, v_j \in C_2, (v_i, v_j) \in E} ((v_i, v_j)) \tag{3.21}$$

A threshold function is used to control the degree to which the difference between components must be larger than minimum internal difference. The pairwise comparison predicate is defined as:

$$D(C_1, C_2) = \begin{cases} true, ifDif(C_1, C_2) > MInt(C_1, C_2) \\ false, otherwise \end{cases} \tag{3.22}$$

where the minimum internal difference Mint is defined as:

$$MInt(C_1, C_2) = \min(Int(C_1) + \tau(C_1), Int(C_2) + \tau(C_2)) \tag{3.23}$$

The threshold function was defined based on the size of the component: $\tau(C) = k/|C|$. The k value is set taking into account the size of the image. For images having the size 128×128, k is set to 150, and for images with size

320×240, k is set to 300. The algorithm for creating the minimum spanning tree can be implemented to run in O (m log m) where m is the number of edges in the graph. The input of the algorithm is represented by a graph $G = (V, E)$ with n vertices and m edges. The obtained output is a segmentation of V in the components $S = (C_1, \ldots, C_r)$. The algorithm has five major steps:

1. Sort E into $\pi = (o_1, \ldots, o_{t\pi})$ by nondecreasing edge weight.
2. Start with a segmentation S^D, where each vertex v_i is in own component.
3. Repeat step 4 for $q = 1, \ldots, m$.
4. Construct S^q using S^{q-1} and the internal difference. If v_i and v_j are in disjoint components of S^{q-1} and the weight of the edge between v_i and v_j is small compared to the internal difference, then merge the two components, otherwise do nothing.
5. Return $S = S^{t\pi}$.

Unlike the classical methods, this technique adaptively adjusts the segmentation criterion based on the degree of variability in neighboring regions of the image.

3.6 Segmentation Error Measures

A potential user of an algorithm's output needs to know what types of incorrect/invalid results to expect, as some types of results might be acceptable while others are not. This called for the use of metrics that are necessary for potential consumers to make intelligent decisions.

This section presents the characteristics of the error metrics defined in [51]. The authors proposed two metrics that can be used to evaluate the consistency of a pair of segmentations, where segmentation is simply a division of the pixels of an image into sets. Thus, a segmentation error measure takes two segmentations $S1$ and $S2$ as input and produces a real valued output in the range [0...1] where zero signifies no error.

The process defines a measure of error at each pixel that is tolerant to refinement as the basis of both measures. A given pixel pi is defined in relation to the segments in $S1$ and 2 that contain that pixel. As the segments are sets of pixels and one segment is a proper subset of the other, then the pixel lies in an area of refinement, and the local error should be zero. If there is no subset relationship, then the two regions overlap in an inconsistent manner. In this case, the local error should be nonzero. Let \ denote set difference and $|x|$ the cardinality of set x. If $R(S; pi)$ is the set of pixels corresponding to the region in segmentation S that contains pixel pi, the local refinement error is defined as in [51]:

$$E(S1, S2, pi) = \frac{|R(S1, pi) \backslash R(S2, pi)|}{|R(S1, pi)|} \tag{3.24}$$

Note that this local error measure is not symmetric. It encodes a measure of refinement in one direction only: $E\ (S1;S2;pi)$ is zero precisely when $S1$ is a refinement of $S2$ at pixel pi, but not vice versa. Given this local refinement error in each direction at each pixel, there are two natural ways to combine the values into an error measure for the entire image. Global consistency error (GCE) forces all local refinements to be in the same direction. Let n be the number of pixels:

$$\mathrm{GCE}(S1,S2)=\frac{1}{n}\min\left\{\sum_i E(S1,S2,pi),\sum_i E(S2,S1,pi),\right\} \tag{3.25}$$

Local Consistency Error (LCE) allows refinement in different directions in different parts of the image.

$$\mathrm{LCE}(S1,S2)=\frac{1}{n}\sum_i \min\{E(S1,S2,pi),E(S2,S1,pi)\} \tag{3.26}$$

As LCE $\leq$ GCE for any two segmentations, it is clear that GCE is a tougher measure than LCE. Martin et al. showed that, as expected, when pairs of human segmentations of the same image are compared, both the GCE and the LCE are low; conversely, when random pairs of human segmentations are compared, the resulting GCE and LCE are high.

3.7 Experiments and Results

This section presents the experimental results for the evaluation of the three segmentation algorithms and error measures values.

The experiments were made on a database with 500 medical images from digestive area captured by an endoscope. The images were taken from patients having diagnoses like: polyps, ulcer, esophagitis, colitis, and ulcerous tumors.

For each image, the following steps are performed by the application that we have created to calculate the GCE and LCE values:

1. Obtain the image regions using the color set back-projection segmentation — CS.
2. Obtain the image regions using the local variation algorithm (LV).
3. Obtain the image regions using the graph-based object detection — GBOD.
4. Obtain the manually segmented regions — MS
5. Store these regions in the database.
6. Calculate GCE and LCE.
7. Store these values in the database for later statistics.

In Table 3.1, the images for which we present some experimental results are presented.

Table 3.1 Images used in experiments

Image Number	
1	2

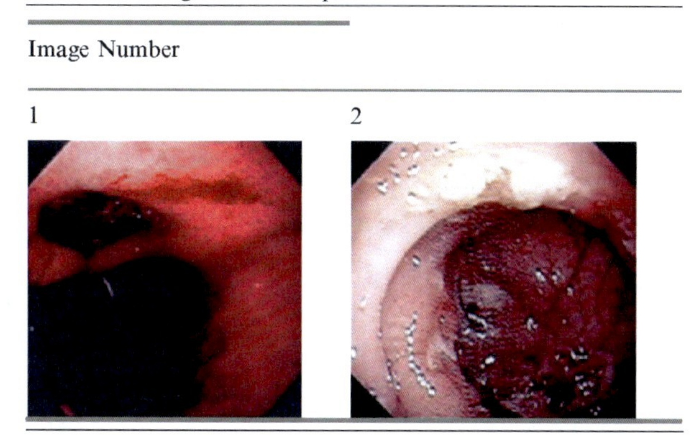

Table 3.2 The number of regions detected for each algorithm

Img. No	CS	LV	GBOD	MS
1	9	5	3	4
2	8	7	2	3

Table 3.3 GCE values calculated for each algorithm

Img. No	GCE-CS	GCE-GBOD	GCE-LV
1	0.18	0.09	0.24
2	0.36	0.10	0.28

Table 3.4 LCE values calculated for each algorithm

Img. No.	LCE-CS	LCE-GBOD	LCE-LV
1	0.11	0.07	0.15
2	0.18	0.12	0.17

In Table 3.2, the number of regions resulted from the application of the segmentation can be seen.

In Table 3.3, the GCE values calculated for each algorithm are presented.

In Table 3.4, the LCE values calculated for each algorithm are presented.

Figures 3.4 and 3.5 present the regions that resulted from manual segmentation and from the application of the three algorithms presented above for images displayed in Table 3.1.

If two different segmentations arise from different perceptual organizations of the scene, then it is fair to declare the segmentations inconsistent. If, however, segmentation is simply a refinement of the other, then the error should be small, or even zero. The error measures presented in the above tables are calculated in relation with the manual segmentation which is considered true segmentation.

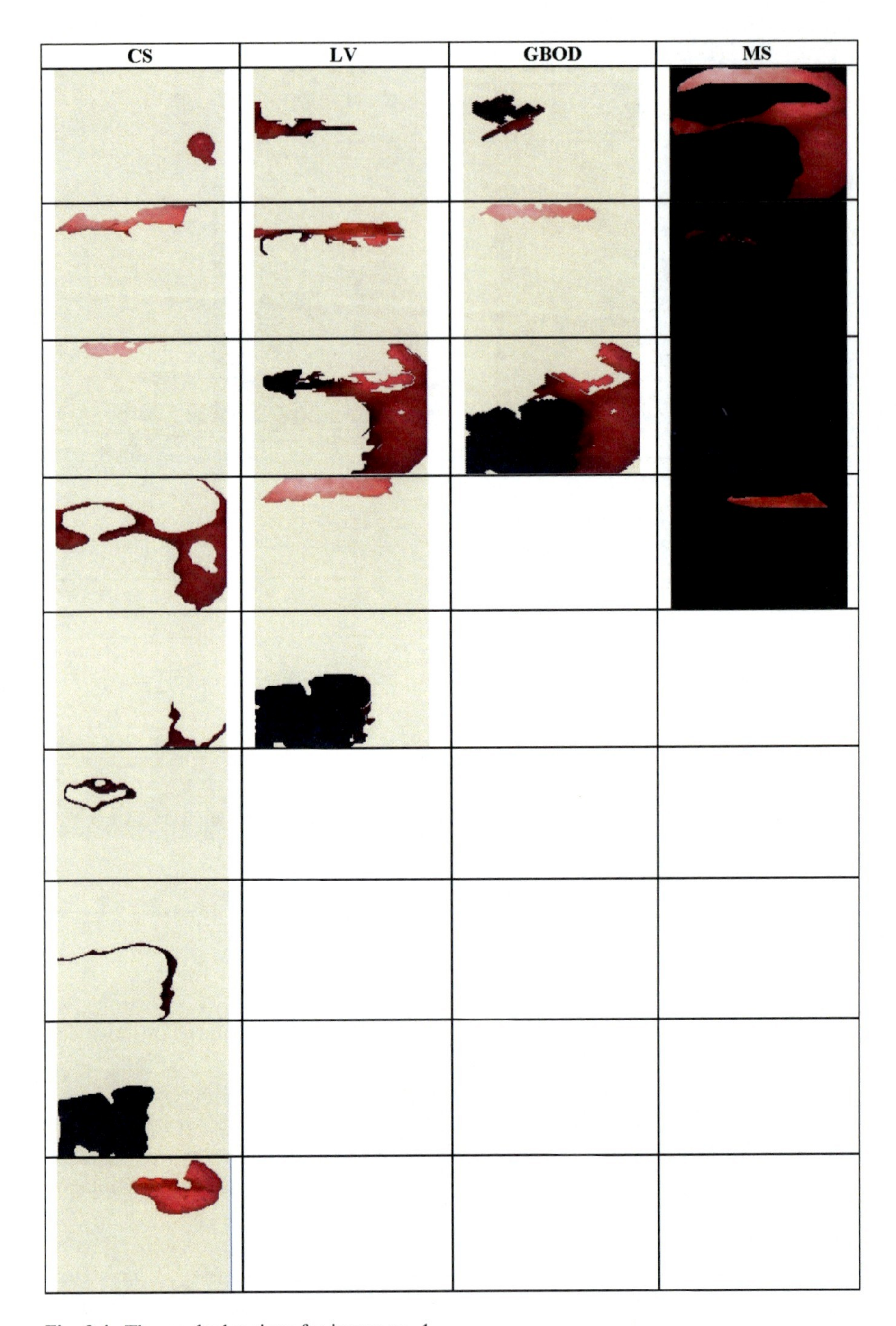

Fig. 3.4 The resulted regions for image no. 1

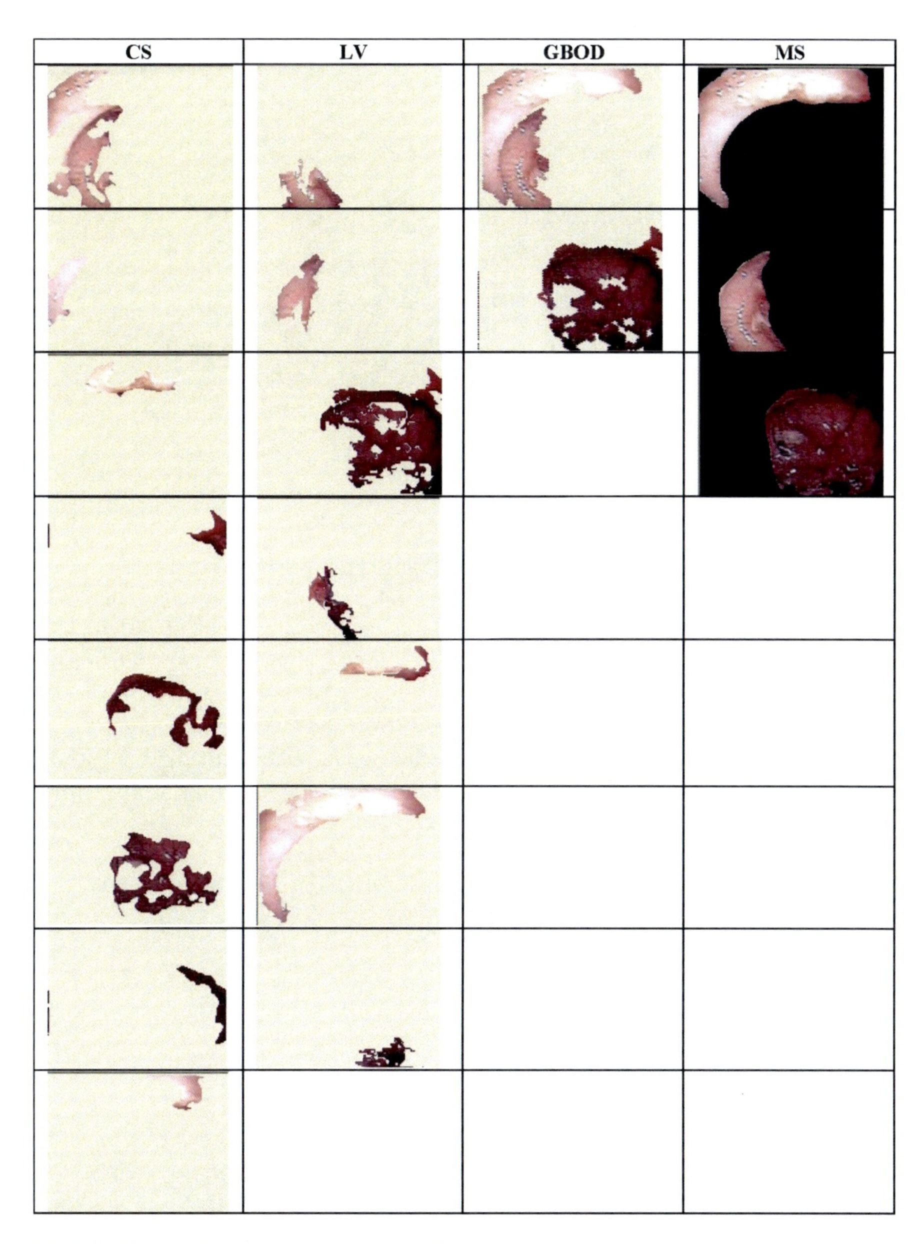

Fig. 3.5 The resulted regions for image no. 2

From the Tables 3.2 and 3.3, it can be observed that the values for GCE and LCE are lower in the case of GBOD method. The error measures, for almost all tested images, have smaller values in the case of the original segmentation method which use a hexagonal structure defined on the set of pixels.

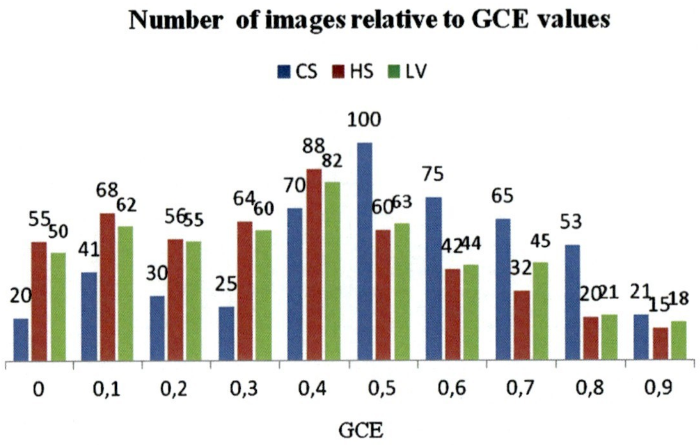

Fig. 3.6 Number of images relative to GCE values

Figure 3.6 presents the repartition of the 500 images from the database repartition on GCE values. The focus point here is the number of images on which the GCE value is under 0.5. In conclusion for GBOD algorithm, a number of 391 images (78%) obtained GCE values under 0.5. Similarly, for CS algorithm, only 286 images (57%) obtained GCE values under 0.5. The segmentation based on LV method is close to our original algorithm: 382 images (76%) had GCE values under 0.5.

Because the error measures for segmentation using GBOD method are lower than for color set back-projection and local variation segmentation, we can infer that the propose segmentation method based on a hexagonal structure is more efficient.

Experimental results show that the original GBOD segmentation method is a good refinement of the manual segmentation.

3.8 Conclusions

This chapter presents an evaluation of three algorithms able to detect regions in endoscopic images: a clustering method (the color set back-projection algorithm), as well as other two methods of segmentation based on graphs: the local variation algorithm and our original segmentation algorithm GBOD.

Our method is based on a hexagonal structure defined on the set of image pixels. The advantage of using a virtual hexagonal network superposed over the initial image pixels is that it reduces the execution time and the memory space used, without losing the initial resolution of the image. In comparison to other segmentation methods, our algorithm is able to adapt and does not require neither parameters for establishing the optimal values nor sets of training images to set parameters.

Firstly, the correctness of segments resulted after the application of the three algorithms described above is compared. Concerning the endoscopic database, all the algorithms have the ability to produce segmentations that comply with the manual segmentation made by a medical expert. Then, for evaluating the accuracy of the segmentation, error measures are used.

The proposed error measures quantify the consistency between segmentations of differing granularities. Because human segmentation is considered true segmentation, the error measures are calculated in relation with manual segmentation. The GCE (global consistency error) and LCE (local consistency error) demonstrate that the graph-based object detection algorithm based on a hexagonal structure produces a better segmentation than the back-projection method and the local variation algorithm.

The future research will focus on developing our segmentation algorithm so as to include the texture feature along with the color feature and reducing the algorithm complexity at $O(n \log n)$, where n represents the number of image pixels.

Referencess

1. Alatan, A., Onural, L., Wollborn, M., Mech, R., Tuncel, E., Sikora, T.: Image sequence analysis for emerging interactive multimedia services-the european cost 211 framework. IEEE Transactions on Circuits and Systems for Video Technology, 8(7), 800–813 (1998)
2. Carson, C., Belongie, S., Greenspan, H., J, J.M.: Blobworld: Color- and texture-based image segmentation using em and its application to image querying and classification. IEEE Transactions on Pattern Analysis and Machine Intelligence, 24(8), 26–37, (2002)
3. Mezaris, V., Kompatsiaris, I., Strintzis, M.: Still image segmentation tools for object-based multimedia applications. International Journal of Pattern Recognition and Artificial Intelligence, 18(4), 700–725 (2004)
4. Fauqueur, J., Boujemaa, N.: Region-based image retrieval: Fast coarse segmentation and fine color description. Journal of Visual Languages and Computing, 15(1), 60–95 (2004)
5. Muller H., Michoux N., Bandon D., Geissbuhler A.: A Review of Content-based Image Retrieval Systems in Medical Application - Clinical Benefits and Future Directions, Int J Med Inform (2004)
6. Pham D.L., Xu C., Prince J.L.: Current methods in medical image segmentation, Annual Review of Biomedical Engineering, 2, 315-337 (2000)
7. Stanescu L., Burdescu D., Brezovan M.: Chapter Book: Multimedia Medical Databases. In: Sidhu, Amandeep S.; Dillon, Tharam; Bellgard, Matthew (Eds.) Biomedical Data and Applications, Series: Studies in Computational Intelligence, 224 (2009)
8. Jiang C., Zhang X., Christoph M.: Hybrid framework for medical image segmentation, Lecture Notes in Computer Science, 3691, 264-271 (2005)
9. Belongie S., Carson C., Greenspan H., Malik J.: Color and Texture-based Image Segmentation Using the Expectation-Maximization Algorithm and Its Application to Content-Based Image Retrieval, ICCV, 675 - 682 (1998)
10. Carson C., Belongie S., Greenspan H., Malik J.: Blobworld: Image segmentation using expectation-maximization and its application to image querying, IEEE Trans. Pattern Analysis and Machine Intelligence, 24(8), 1026-1038 (2002)
11. Ballerini L.: Medical image segmentation using Genetic snakes, Applications and science of neural networks, fuzzy systems, and evolutionary computation II, Denver Co (1999)

12. Ghebreab S., Smeulders A.W.M.: Medical Images Segmentation by Strings, Proceedings of the VISIM Workshop: Information Retrieval and Exploration in Large Collections of Medical Images (2001)
13. Ghebreab S., Smeulders A.W.M.: An approximately complete string representation of local object boundary features for concept-based image retrieval, IEEE International Symposium on Biomedical Imaging (2004)
14. Gordon S., Zimmerman G., Greenspan H.: Image segmentation of uterine cervix images for indexing in PACS, Proceedings of the 17th IEEE Symposium on Computer-Based Medical Systems, CBMS (2004)
15. Lamecker H., Lange T., Seeba M., Eulenstein S., Westerhoff M., Hege H.C.: Automatic Segmentation of the Liver for Preoperative Planning of Resections, Proceedings of Medicine Meets Virtual Reality, Studies in Health Technologies and Informatics, 94, 171-174 (2003)
16. Muller H., Marquis S., Cohen G., Poletti P.A., Lovis C.L., Geissbuhler A.: Automatic abnormal region detection in lung CT images for visual retrieval, Swiss Medical Informatics, 57, 2-6 (2005)
17. Felzenszwalb, P., Huttenlocher, W. : Efficient graph-based image segmentation. International Journal of Computer Vision, 59(2), 167–181 (2004)
18. Guigues, L., Herve, L., Cocquerez, L.P.: The hierarchy of the cocoons of a graph and its application to image segmentation. Pattern Recognition Letters, 24(8), 1059–1066 (2003).
19. Shi, J., Malik, J.: Normalized cuts and image segmentation. IEEE Transactions on Pattern Analysis and Machine Intelligence, 22(8), 885–905 (2000)
20. Wu, Z., Leahy, R.: An optimal graph theoretic approach to data clustering: theory and its application to image segmentation. IEEE Transactions on Pattern Analysis and Machine Intelligence, 15(11), 1101–1113 (1993)
21. Zahn, C.: Graph-theoretical methods for detecting and describing gestal clusters. IEEE Transactions on Computers, 20(1), 68–86 (1971)
22. Urquhar, R.: Graph theoretical clustering based on limited neighborhood sets. Pattern Recognition, 15(3), 173–187 (1982).
23. Gdalyahu, Y., Weinshall, D., Werman, M.: Self-organization in vision: stochastic clustering for image segmentation, perceptual grouping, and image database organization. IEEE Transactions on Pattern Analysis and Machine Intelligence, 23(10), 1053–1074. (2001)
24. Jermyn, I., Ishikawa, H.: Globally optimal regions and boundaries as minimum ratio weight cycles. IEEE Transactions on Pattern Analysis and Machine Intelligence, 23(8), 1075–1088 (2001)
25. Cooper, M.: The tractibility of segmentation and scene analysis. International Journal of Computer Vision, 30(1), 27–42 (1998)
26. Pavlidis, T.: Structural Pattern Recognition. New York: Springer Verlag (1977)
27. Malik, J., Belongie, S., Leung, T., Shi, J.: Contour and texture analysis for image segmentation. International Journal of Computer Vision, 43(1), 7–27(2001)
28. Comaniciu, D., Meer, P.: Robust analysis of feature spaces: color image segmentation. IEEE Transactions on Pattern Analysis and Machine Intelligence, 24(5), 603–619 (2002)
29. Jain, A., Dubes, R.: Algorithms for clustering data. Englewood, NJ.: Prentice Hall (1988)
30. Comaniciu, D., Meer, P.: Mean shift analysis and applications. In Proceedings of the IEEE Conference on Computer Vision and Pattern Recognition, Madison, Wisconsin, 1197–1203 (1999)
31. Garrido, L., Salembier, P.: Region based analysis of video sequences with a general merging algorithm. Proceedings of the European Signal Processing Conference (EUSIPCO), Rhodes, Greece, 1697–1700 (1998)
32. Bennstrom, C., Casas, J.: Binary-partition-tree creation using a quasi-inclusion criterion. In Proceedings of the Eighth International Conference on Information Visualization, London, UK, pp. 259–294 (2004)
33. Huang, T.-H., Cheng, K.-Y., Chuang, Y.-Y.: A collaborative benchmark for region of interest detection algorithms. In Proceedings of the International Conference on Computer Vision and Pattern Recognition, Miami Beach, USA, 296–303 (2009)

34. Achanta, R.: Frequency-tuned Salient Region Detection - Ground Truth Used for Comparison (2009) http: //ivrg.epfl.ch/supplementary_material/RK_ . Acessed 26 July 2011
35. Cao, G., Cheikh, F.-A.: Salient Region Detection with Opponent Color Boosting. Processings of the European Workshop on Visual Information, Paris, France, 13–18 (2010)
36. Donoser, M., Bischof, H. ROI-SEG: Unsupervised Color Segmentation by Combining Differently Focused Sub Results. Proceedings of the IEEE Conference on Computer Vision and Pattern Recognition, Minneapolis, SUA, 1–8 (2007).
37. Liu, T., Sun, J., Zheng, N.-N., Tang, X., Shum, H.-Y.: Learning to Detect A Salient Object. Proceedings of the IEEE International Conference on Computer Vision and pattern Recognition, Minneapolis, Minnesota, 1–8 (2007)
38. Burdescu, D.D., Brezovan M., Ganea, E., Stanescu L.: A New Method for Segmentation of Images Represented in a HSV Color Space. ACIVS 2009, 606-617(2009)
39. Burdescu, D.D., Brezovan M., Ganea E., Stanescu L.: New Algorithm for Segmentation of Images Represented as Hypergraph Hexagonal-Grid. IbPRIA 2011, 395-402 (2011)
40. Brezovan, M., Burdescu, D., Ganea, E., Stanescu, L.: An Adaptive Method for Efficient Detection of Salient Visual Object from Color Images. Proceedings of the 20th International Conference on Pattern Recognition, Istambul, Turkey, 2346–2349 (2010)
41. Brezovan, M., Burdescu, D., Ganea, E., Stanescu, L.: A new method for segmentation of images represented in a HSV color space. Lecture Notes in Computer Science, 5807, 606–616 (2009)
42. Adamek, T., O'Connor, N.,Murphy, N.: Region-based segmentation of images using syntactic visual features. Proceedings of the International Workshop on Image Analysis for Multimedia Interactive Services (WIAMIS '05), Montreux, Switzerland (2005)
43. Gonzales, R., Wintz, P.: Digital Image Processing. Reading, MA: Addison-Wesley (1987).
44. He, X., jia, W.: Hexagonal Structure for Intelligent Vision. Proceedings of The First International Conference on Information and Technologies, Karachi, Pakistan, 52-64 (2005)
45. Middleton, L., Sivaswamy, J.: Hexagonal Image Processing; A Practical Approach (Advances in Pattern Recognition). Springer-Verlag (2005)
46. Staunton, R.C.: The design of hexagonal sampling structures for image digitization and their use with local operators. Image Vision Computing, 7(3), 162–166 (1989)
47. Billmeyer, F., Salzman,M.: Principles of color technology. New York: Wiley (1981)
48. Cormen, T., Leiserson, C., Rivest, R.: Introduction to algorithms. Cambridge, MA: MIT Press (1990)
49. Smith, J.R., Chang, S.F.: Tools and Techniques for Color Image Retrieval. Science and Technology - Storage & Retrieval for Image and Video Databases IV, 2670, San Jose, CA, February 1996. IS&T/SPIE (1996)
50. Pantofaru C., Hebert, M.: A Comparison of Image Segmentation Algorithms. Technical Report CMU-RI-TR-05-40, Robotics Institute, Carnegie Mellon University, Pittsburgh, Pennsylvania (2005)
51. Martin D., Fowlkes, C., Tal, D., Malik, J.: A Database of Human Segmented Natural Images and its Application to Evaluating Segmentation Algorithms and Measuring Ecological Statistics, *IEEE (ed.), Proceedings of the Eighth International Conference On Computer Vision (ICCV-01)*, Vancouver, British Columbia, Canada, vol. 2, July 2001, 416–425

Chapter 4
Ontologies

4.1 Ontologies: A General Overview

The term ontology originated as a science within philosophy but evolved over time being used in various domains of computer science during the 1990s by several Artificial Intelligence (AI) research communities. It has recently been used in several other information technology fields such as intelligent information integration, information retrieval on the Internet, and knowledge management. Ontologies are of basic interest in many different fields because they provide a shared and common understanding of some domain that can be the basis for communication ground across the gaps between people and computers [1].

Ontologies are enabling knowledge sharing and support for external reasoning. Ontologies can be used for improving the process of information retrieval, for solving the problem of heterogeneous information sources that utilize different representations, to analyze, model, and implement the domain knowledge. A taxonomy represents a classification of the data in a domain. Ontology is different than taxonomy from two important perspectives: it has a richer internal structure as it includes relations and constraints between the concepts, and it claims to represent a certain consensus about the knowledge in the domain. This consensus is among the intended users of the knowledge, for example, doctors using a hospital ontology regarding a certain disease. Computational ontologies are a means to formally model the structure of a system, the relevant entities, and relations that emerge from its observation [2]. The ontology engineer analyzes relevant entities and organizes them into concepts and relations, being represented, respectively, by unary and binary predicates. The backbone of an ontology consists of a generalization/specialization hierarchy of concepts, a taxonomy. Ontologies can be very useful in improving the semantic information retrieval process by allowing an abstractization and an explicit representation of the information. Ontologies can possess inference functions, allowing more intelligent retrieval.

An ontology represents an explicit and formal specification of a conceptualization [3] containing a finite list of relevant terms and the relationships between them.

L. Stanescu et al., *Creating New Medical Ontologies for Image Annotation: A Case Study*, SpringerBriefs in Electrical and Computer Engineering,
DOI 10.1007/978-1-4614-1909-9_4,

A "conceptualization" is an abstract model of a phenomenon, created by identification of the relevant concepts of the phenomenon. The concepts, the relations between them, and the constraints on their use are explicitly defined. "Formal" means that ontology is machine-readable and excludes the use of natural languages. In medical domains, the concepts are diseases and symptoms, the relations between them are causal, and a constraint is that a disease cannot cause itself. A "shared conceptualization" means that ontologies aim to represent consensual knowledge intended for the use of a group.

A taxonomy represents a classification of the data in a domain. The difference between a taxonomy and an ontology concerns two important contexts: an ontology has a richer internal structure because it contains the relations and constraints between the concept, and an ontology claims to represent a certain consensus about the knowledge in the domain.

In [4], an ontology is a formal explicit description of concepts in a domain of discourse (classes sometimes called concepts), properties of each concept describing various features and attributes of the concept (slots sometimes called roles or properties), and restrictions on slots (facets sometimes called role restrictions). Classes are the focus of most ontologies. Classes describe concepts in the domain, and slots describe properties of classes and instances. From practical point of view, the development of an ontology includes: defining classes in the ontology, arranging the classes in a taxonomic (subclass–superclass) hierarchy, defining slots, and describing allowed values for these slots, filling in the values for slots for instances.

Ontologies have a dominant role in a high number of different fields like:

(a) Natural language applications—being used for:

- *Natural language processing* (Generalized Upper Model [5], SENSUS [6]). The Generalized Upper Model is a general task and domain independent "linguistically motivated ontology" that provides semantics for natural language expressions. The categories of the ontology enforce a consistent modeling style on any domain which is also guaranteedly appropriate for flexible expression in natural language. SENSUS is a 70,000-node terminology taxonomy and a framework into which additional knowledge can be placed. SENSUS is an extension and reorganization of WordNet at the top level containing nodes from the Penman Upper Model [7], and the major branches of WordNet have been rearranged to fit.
- *Automatic extraction of knowledge from scientific texts* (Plinius Ontology [8]). The Plinius ontology of ceramic materials covers the conceptualization of the chemical composition of materials. The ontology of ceramic materials is given as a conceptual construction kit, involving several sets of atomic concepts and construction rules for making complex concepts.
- *WordNet* is one of the largest lexical Ontologies.

(b) *Database and information retrieval*—being used for:

- Improving the process of retrieval
- Solving the problem of heterogeneous information sources that utilize different representations
- Intraorganization communication and knowledge management

(c) *Knowledge engineering*—being used for analyzing, modeling, and implementing the domain knowledge, but also affecting problem-solving knowledge.

According to their level of generality, ontologies can also be categorized in two main classes [1]:

(a) Ontologies that capture "static knowledge" about a domain:

- *Domain ontologies*—designed to represent knowledge relevant to a certain domain type, for example, medical, mechanical, etc.
- *Generic ontologies*—can be applied to a variety of domain types, for example, technical domains.
- *Representational ontologies*—these formulate general representation entities without defining what should be represented, for example, frame ontology [9].

(b) Ontologies that provide a reasoning point of view about the domain knowledge (problem-solving knowledge).

- *Task ontologies*—provide terms specific for particular tasks
- *Method ontologies*—provide terms specific to particular problem-solving methods

A distinct type of ontology is represented by *Application Ontologies* representing a combination of the Domain and Method Ontologies.

4.2 Ontology Design and Development Tools

For an ontology design process, three fundamental rules should be taken into account:

1. There is no one correct way to model a domain—there are always viable alternatives.
2. Ontology development is necessarily an iterative process.
3. Concepts in the ontology should be close to objects (physical or logical) and relationships in the domain of interest.

In [10], a set of design criteria for ontologies whose purpose is knowledge sharing and interoperation among programs based on a shared conceptualization is proposed:

(a) *Clarity*—an ontology should effectively communicate the intended meaning of defined terms, and the definitions should be objective.
(b) *Coherence*—an ontology should be coherent. This means that it should sanction inferences that are consistent with the definitions. The defining axioms should be logically consistent. Coherence should also apply to the concepts that are defined informally, such as those described in natural language documentation and examples.
(c) *Extendibility*—an ontology should be designed to anticipate the uses of the shared vocabulary. It should be possible to define new terms for special uses based on the existing vocabulary, in a way that does not require the revision of the existing definitions.
(d) *Minimal encoding bias*—the conceptualization should be specified at the knowledge level without depending on a particular symbol-level encoding. An encoding bias results when a representation choices are made purely for the convenience of notation or implementation and should be minimized because knowledge-sharing agents may be implemented in different representation systems and styles of representation.
(e) *Minimal ontological commitment*—an ontology should require the minimal ontological commitment sufficient to support the intended knowledge sharing activities. An ontology should make as few claims as possible about the world being modeled, allowing the parties committed to the ontology freedom to specialize and instantiate the ontology as needed.

A general process of iterative design used to obtain an ontology contains several steps:

(a) *Determining the domain and the scope of the ontology*—to define the domain and the scope, a response should be given to the following questions: what is the domain covered by the ontology? For what purpose will the ontology be used? In our case, the domain is represented by medical domain, and the ontology is used for the annotation process.
(b) *Reusing existing ontologies*—it is a good approach to consider what someone else has done and to check if something can be refined and if existing sources for our particular domain and task can be extended. Reusing existing ontologies can be a requirement if the system needs to interact with other applications that have already committed to particular ontologies or controlled vocabularies. Existing ontologies like Open Biological and Biomedical Ontologies can have formats that are not always easy to interpret. For this reason, we have decided to create a custom ontology.
(c) *Enumerating important terms in the ontology*—it is useful to write down a list of all terms we would like either to make statements about or to explain to a user. What are the terms we would like to talk about? What properties do those

terms have? What would we like to say about those terms? The descriptors provided by MeSH are representing the terms that should be taken into account.

(d) *Defining the classes and the class hierarchy*—there are several possible approaches in developing a class hierarchy [11]:

- *A top-down development process* starts with the definition of the most general concepts in the domain and subsequent specialization of the concepts.
- *A bottom-up development process* starts with the definition of the most specific classes, the leaves of the hierarchy, with subsequent grouping of these classes into more general concepts.
- *A combination development process* is a combination of the top-down and bottom-up approaches. We have used a top-down development process for our ontology. The following classes were identified: *concept*, *hierarchical*, *child*, and *parent*.

(e) *Defining the properties of classes (slots)*—once we have defined some of the classes, we must describe the internal structure of concepts. For example, the fields associated with a descriptor will be used to define the properties of the *concept* class.

(f) *Defining the facets of the slots*—slots can have different facets describing the value type, allowed values, the number of the values (cardinality), and other features of the values the slot can take.

(g) *Creating instances*—the last step is creating individual instances of classes in the hierarchy. Defining an individual instance of a class requires choosing a class, creating an individual instance of that class, and filling in the slot values. Each descriptor will be represented as an instance of the *concept* class, and each hierarchical relationship existing between any two descriptors will be represented as an instance of the *hierarchical* class.

There is a great variety of development tools for ontologies including:

- *Protégé* 3.2 [12] is a version of the Protégé OWL editor [13] created by the Stanford Medical Informatics group at Stanford University. Protégé is a Java-based open-source standalone application to be installed and run a local computer. It enables users to load and save OWL [14] and RDF [15] ontologies, edit and visualize classes and properties, define logical class characteristics as OWL expressions, and edit OWL individuals. With respect to the supported languages, Protégé is a hybrid tool. The internal storage format of Protégé is frame-based. Reasoning can be performed by means of an API which employs an external DIG (a standardized XML interface to Description Logics systems) [16] compliant reasoner, such as RACER [17], FaCT++ [18], or KAON2 [19].
- *Altova SemanticWorks*™ is a commercial OWL editor offered by Altova. The most outstanding feature of the tool is the graphical interface, and it supports the visual editing of OWL and RDF(S) files using a rich, graph-based multidocument user interface. The latter supports various graphical elements including connections and compartments. The visualization of ontologies

utilizes very similar mechanisms from the other Altova products, which are XML-based. The strength of SemanticWorks™ is the graphical interface with its navigation capabilities.

- *TopBraid Composer*™ is a modeling tool for the creation and maintenance of ontologies. It is a complete editor for RDF(S) and OWL models. TopBraid Composer™ is built upon the Eclipse platform and uses Jena [20] as its underlying API. The following list contains some of the characteristics of the tool. It is implemented as an IDE application using the Eclipse platform with all its advantages (such as the plug-in concept). TopBraid Composer™ supports consistency checks and other reasoning tasks. The system has the open-source DL reasoner Pellet built-in as its default inference engine, but other classifiers can be accessed via the DIG interface.
- *IODT* Integrated Ontology Development Toolkit (IODT) was developed by IBM. This toolkit includes the Ontology Definition Metamodel (EODM), EODM workbench, and an OWL Ontology Repository (named Minerva). EODM is derived from the OMG's Ontology Definition Metamodel (ODM) and implemented in Eclipse Modeling Framework (EMF). The EODM workbench is an Eclipse-based editor for users to create, view, and generate OWL ontologies. It has UML-like graphic notions to represent OWL class, restriction and property, etc. The EODM workbench supports multiple views for ontologies, enabling users to visually split large models. These views are independent from each other but synchronized automatically.
- *SWOOP* [21] is an open-source hypermedia-based OWL ontology editor. The user interface design of SWOOP follows a browser paradigm, including the typical navigation features like history buttons. Offering an environment with a look and feel known from Web browsers, the developers of swoop aimed at a concept that average users are expected to accept within short time. Thus, users are enabled to view and edit OWL ontologies in a "Web-like" manner, which concerns the navigation via hyperlinks but also annotation features.
- *OntoStudio*® is a commercial product of Ontoprise. It is the front-end counterpart to OntoBroker®, a fast datalog-based F-Logic inference machine. Consequently, a focus of the OntoStudio® development has been on the support of various tasks around the application of rules. This includes the direct creation of rules (via a graphical rule editor) but also the application of rules for the dynamic integration of data sources (using a database schema import and a mapping tool). OntoStudio® offers a graphical and a textual rule editor as well as debugging features as well as a form-based query editor. It also includes a graphical editor for the creation and management of ontology mappings including conditional mappings, filters, and transformations.

4.3 Medical Ontologies

The main goal of using ontologies in the medical domain is that of representation and reorganization of medical terminologies. Building ontologies for representing medical terminology systems is a difficult task that requires a profound analysis of the structure and the concepts of medical terms, but necessary in order to solve situations that appear frequently in medical life. So, medical stuff developed their own specialized languages and lexicons used to store and communicate general medical knowledge and patient-related information in an efficient manner. Such terminologies are optimized for human processing and contain a significant amount of implicit knowledge. Medical information systems, on the other hand, need to be able to communicate complex and detailed medical concepts (possibly expressed in different languages) without ambiguity. We can find also ontology-based applications in the field of Medical Natural Language Processing.

The benefits of using medical ontologies are:

- Possibly, the most significant benefit that ontologies may bring to healthcare systems is their ability to support the integration of knowledge and data that is very necessary.
- Ontologies can be the base for building more powerful and more interoperable information systems in healthcare.
- Ontologies can support processes like transmitting, reusing, and sharing patient data that are important in healthcare.
- Ontologies can provide semantic-based criteria for computing different statistical aggregations.

As a negative aspect, some remain skeptical about the impact that ontologies may have on the design and maintenance of real-world healthcare information systems.

Some of the important projects on medical ontologies will be described next.

GALEN (**G**eneralized **A**rchitecture for **L**anguages, **E**ncyclopedias, and **N**omenclatures in medicine) was concerned with the computerization of clinical terminologies in order to satisfy the next two aspects [22]:

- Allow clinical information to be captured, represented, manipulated, and displayed in a more powerful way.
- Support reuse of information to integrate medical records, decision support, and other clinical systems. As a result, GALEN replaces the static hierarchy of traditional clinical terminologies with a description logic.

Traditional terminologies, optimized for direct human use, cannot satisfy our hopes for extensive data analysis, sharing, and reuse. New kinds of terminology, designed for computation, are required. The GALEN project proposed to replace the monolithic static lookup terminologies with a common reference model (ontology) that can be dynamically extended using an automatic classification engine, in a terminology server.

The main components of the GALEN projects are [22]:

- The GALEN Representation and Integration Language (GRAIL) Kernel which is a fully compositional and generative formal system for modeling concepts. It also provides a separation between the concept model and linguistic mechanisms which interpret that model in order to allow the development of multilingual systems.
- A Coding Reference (CORE) Model of medical terminology covering was developed which aims to represent the core concepts in, for example, pathology, anatomy, and therapeutics that have widespread applicability in medical applications.
- A Terminology Server (TeS) which encapsulates and coordinates the functionality of the concept module, multilingual module, and code conversion module. It also provides a uniform applications programming interface and network services for use by external applications.

The GALEN vision of computed ontologies has been adopted, adapted, and developed in other domains like bioinformatics.

ONIONS (**ON**tological **I**ntegration **O**f **N**aive **S**ources) **project** had as a main goal the developing of a large-scale ontology library for medical terminology. The developed methodology uses a description logic-based design for the modules in the library and generic theories, creating in this way a stratification of the modules. By conceptual analysis and ontology integration over a set of authoritative sources, the terminological knowledge is obtained [23].

The purposes of ONIONS are [23]:

- Developing a set of generic ontologies to be the base for the conceptual integration of important ontologies in medicine.
- Making a set of relevant domain ontologies fits in a formally and conceptually satisfactory ontology library to allow the execution of several tasks such as information access and retrieval, digital content integration, computerized guidelines generation, etc.
- The possibility of following the steps of the procedure of building an ontology, therefore making its maintenance (evaluation, extensions and/or updating, and intersubjective consensus) easier.

The main components of the ONIONS project are [23]:

- ON9.2 ontology library
- The IMO (Integrated Medical Ontology) that represents the integration of five medical top levels of relevant terminologies and the relative mappings
- A formalized representation of some medical repositories (mainly the UMLS Metathesaurus™ defined by the US National Library of Medicine) with their classification within the IMO

The main purpose of the Medical Ontology Research program from *Lister Hill National Center for Biomedical Communications* [24] is developing a strong medical ontology to allow communication between various knowledge processing applications.

The steps for creating a usable ontology are [24]:

- *Definition*—Semantic information which is being provided by existing terminologies, knowledge bases, expert systems, or extracted from the medical literature defines the semantic spaces.
- *Organization*—In order to organize the semantic spaces, semantic networks can be used.
- *Visualization*—Users can visualize the semantic spaces after they have been defined and organized. This visualization helps users navigate to the information they seek. Problems like granularity, redundancy, and consistency between sources must be solved before designing applications for the visualization and navigation of semantic spaces.
- *Utilization*—Semantic spaces deliver the basic knowledge used in applications like concept-based indexing, concept-based retrieval, and terminology servers by specifying relationships of proximity between concepts.

This ontology uses the next primary knowledge sources: UMLS, SNOMED-RT, GALEN, MEDLINE citations, medical encyclopedias, and medical corpora.

It will assist other National Library of Medicine projects for providing a well organized and more complete representation of their biomedical information.

The *Gene Ontology* (GO) represents an important bioinformatics project with the goal of standardizing the representation of gene and gene product attributes across species and databases [25, 26].

The GO project is a collaborative one, starting with relation between three model organism databases, FlyBase (*Drosophila*), the *Saccharomyces* Genome Database (SGD), and the Mouse Genome Database (MGD), in 1998. In time, the GO Consortium has expended and now includes many databases with data about plant, animal, and microbial genomes.

The project provides a controlled vocabulary of terms for describing gene product characteristics and gene product annotation data from GO Consortium members. The GO project also provides the necessary tools to access and process this data.

The ontology covers three domains: cellular component, molecular function, and biological process [25, 26].

The GO ontology is built as a directed acyclic graph, and each term has defined relationships to one or more other terms in the same domain and sometimes to other domains. The GO vocabulary is designed to be species neutral and includes terms applicable to prokaryotes and eukaryotes, single and multicellular organisms.

The project consists of three different parts:

1. The development and maintenance of the ontologies.
2. The annotation of gene products.
3. The development of tools that facilitate the creation, maintenance, and use of ontologies.

Another example is the *Foundational Model of Anatomy* ontology (FMA) [27]. FMA is a domain ontology created to represent a coherent body of explicit declarative knowledge about human anatomy. This ontological framework can be applied and extended to all other species. This ontology represents in a symbolic way the phenotypic structure of the human body in a form that is understandable to humans and is also navigable, parseable, and interpretable by machine-based systems. This symbolic representation uses classes or types and relationships.

The FMA ontology is integrated in the distributed framework of the Anatomy Information System developed and maintained by the Structural Informatics Group at the University of Washington.

The Foundational Model of Anatomy ontology consists of four components that are closely related [27]:

- *Anatomy taxonomy* (At) classifies anatomical entities according to the characteristics they share (genus) and by which they make the difference between each other (differentia).
- *Anatomical Structural Abstraction* (ASA) specifies the relationships of type part-whole and spatial that exist between the entities represented in At.
- *Anatomical Transformation Abstraction* (ATA) points out the morphological transformation of the entities represented in At during prenatal development and the postnatal life cycle.
- *Metaknowledge* (Mk) specifies the principles, rules, and definitions taken into consideration at the representation of classes and relationships in the other three components of FMA.

It can be said that the Foundational Model of Anatomy ontology may be represented by the abstraction [27]:

$$\text{FMA} = (\text{At, ASA, ATA, Mk})$$

4.4 Topic Maps

Topic Maps [28] is an ISO standard for the representation and interchange of knowledge, with an emphasis on the findability of information. The standard is formally known as ISO/IEC 13250:2003. A Topic Map can represent information using *topics*—representing concepts, *associations*—representing the relationships between topics, and *occurrences*—representing relationships between topics and information resources relevant to them. Topics, associations, and occurrences can be typed, but the types must be defined by the creator of the Topic Map, and is known as the ontology of the topic map.

Topic Maps have a standard XML-based interchange syntax called XML Topic Maps (XTM) [29]. A format called Linear Topic Map notation (LTM) [30] serves as a kind of shorthand for writing Topic Maps in plain text editors. This is useful for writing short personal topic maps or exchange partial topic maps by e-mail. This format can be converted to XTM. There is another format called AsTMa [31] which serves a similar purpose. When writing Topic Maps manually, it is much more compact, but of course can be converted to XTM.

Topic Maps were originally designed to handle the construction of indexes, glossaries, thesauri, and tables of contents, but their applicability extends beyond that domain. They can serve to represent information currently stored as database schemas (relational and object). Where databases only capture the relations between information objects, Topic Maps also allow these objects to be connected to the various places where they occur. Topic Maps render information assets independent of software applications. The high-level nature of Topic Maps makes them attractive to information architects, who need powerful means of representing a virtually unlimited number of relationship types between a virtually unlimited numbers of information types. Topic Maps encompass a whole range of knowledge representation schemas, from very straightforward and unambiguous to quite complex and even ambiguous information. It is highly desirable for representing relationships that may be true or false, depending on circumstance.

The terminology used by the XTM syntax to describe documents includes the following elements:

1. *Association*—a relationship between topics represented by an XML element named < *association* >.
2. *Association type*—one of the association classes specified for the < *association* > element using the < instanceOf > element.
3. *Member*—is represented by the < member > XML element and is defined as a child of the < *association* > element.
4. *Role*—represents the role played by a topic item as a member of an association.
5. *Topic Map*—represents a collection of topics, associations, and scopes but also the < topicmap > XML element of a Topic Map document defined using the XTM syntax.
6. *Topic Map document*—a document containing one or more Topic Maps.
7. *Occurrence*—a child element (<occurrence>) of a < topic > element.
8. *Occurrence type*—one of the classes of topic occurrence. The class of topic occurrence is specified by an < occurrence > element's < instanceOf > child element.
9. *Topic*—a resource that acts as a proxy for some subject being represented by the < topic > element.

Topic Maps provide a bridge between the domains of knowledge representation and information management. Topics and associations build a networked information overlay above information resources that allows users to navigate at a higher level of abstraction. Topic Maps are very powerful in their ability to organize information, but they may be very large. Because of this several visualization, techniques like Ontopia Navigator [32], Empolis K42 [33], TM4L [34], etc. were developed.

4.5 MeSH Description

Medical Subject Headings (MeSH) [35] is a comprehensive controlled vocabulary for the purpose of indexing journal articles and books in the life sciences; it can also serve as a thesaurus that facilitates searching. Created and updated by the US

National Library of Medicine (NLM), it is used by the MEDLINE/PubMed article database and by NLM's catalog of book holdings. In MEDLINE/PubMed, every journal article is indexed with some 10–15 headings or subheadings, with one or two of them designated as *major* and marked with an asterisk. When performing a MEDLINE search via PubMed, entry terms are automatically translated into the corresponding descriptors. The Medical Subject Headings staffs continually revise and update the MeSH vocabulary. Staff subject specialists are responsible for areas of the health sciences in which they have knowledge and expertise. MeSH's structure contains a high number of subject headings also known as descriptors. Most of these are accompanied by a short description or definition, links to related descriptors, and a list of synonyms or very similar terms known as *entry terms*. Because of these synonym lists, MeSH can also be viewed as a thesaurus. The *descriptors* or *subject headings* are arranged in a hierarchy, and a given descriptor may appear at several places in the hierarchical tree. The tree numbers indicate the places within the MeSH hierarchies, also known as the Tree Structures, in which the MH appears. Thus, the numbers are the formal computable representation of the hierarchical relationships. The tree locations carry systematic labels known as *tree numbers*, and one descriptor may have several tree numbers. For example, the descriptor "digestive system neoplasms" has the tree numbers C06.301 and C04.588.274. The tree numbers of a given descriptor are subject to change as MeSH is updated. Every descriptor also carries a unique alphanumerical ID called *DescriptorUI* that will not change.

Two important relationship types are defined for MeSH content: hierarchical relationships and associative relationships [36]. The hierarchical relationships are fundamental components in a thesaurus, and MeSH has long formalized its hierarchical structure in an extensive tree structure, currently at nine levels, representing increasing levels of specificity. This structure enables browsing for the appropriately specific descriptor. Many examples of hierarchical relations are instances of the part-whole and class-subclass relationships, which are relatively well understood. Since its hierarchical relationships are between descriptors, a MeSH descriptor can have different children in different trees. Hierarchical relationships in the MeSH thesaurus are at the level of the descriptor. Hierarchical relationships are seen as parent–child relationships. Associative relationships are used to point out in the thesaurus, the existence of other descriptors, which may be more appropriate for a particular purpose. They may point out distinctions made in the thesaurus or in the way the thesaurus has arranged descriptors hierarchically. Many associative relationships are represented by the "see related" cross-reference. The categories of relationships seem to be greater in number and are certainly more varied than hierarchical relationships. One attribute which can be thought of as an associative relationship within the MeSH thesaurus is the pharmacologic action. Limited to chemicals, this relationship allows the aggregation of chemicals by actions or uses. MeSH content that can be obtained from [37] and is offered as an XML file named desc2010.xml (2010 version) containing the descriptors and a txt file named mtrees2010.txt containing the hierarchical structure.

```
<DescriptorRecord DescriptorClass = "1">
     <DescriptorUI>D003092</DescriptorUI>
     <DescriptorName>
        <String>Colitis</String>
     </DescriptorName>
        <TreeNumberList>
        <TreeNumber>C06.405.205.265</TreeNumber>
       <TreeNumber>C06.405.469.158.188</TreeNumber>
   </TreeNumberList>
 </DescriptorRecord>

<DescriptorRecord DescriptorClass = "1">
    <DescriptorUI>D003093</DescriptorUI>
      <DescriptorName>
       <String>Colitis, Ulcerative</String>
      </DescriptorName>
   <TreeNumberList>
    <TreeNumber>C06.405.205.265.231</TreeNumber>
    <TreeNumber>C06.405.205.731.249</TreeNumber>
    <TreeNumber>C06.405.469.158.188.231</TreeNumber>
    <TreeNumber>C06.405.469.432.249</TreeNumber>
   </TreeNumberList>
</DescriptorRecord>
```

Fig. 4.1 Reduced representation of two MeSH descriptors

```
Esophageal Diseases;C06.405.117
    Esophageal Atresia;C06.405.117.260
    Esophageal Cyst;C06.405.117.316
    Esophageal Fistula;C06.405.117.367
        Tracheoesophageal Fistula;C06.405.117.367.725
    Esophageal Neoplasms;C06.405.117.430
    Esophageal Perforation;C06.405.117.468
        Mallory-Weiss Syndrome;C06.405.117.468.524
    Esophageal Stenosis;C06.405.117.544
    Esophagitis;C06.405.117.620
        Esophagitis, Peptic;C06.405.117.620.420
Gastroenteritis;C06.405.205
    Appendicitis;C06.405.205.099
    Cholera Morbus;C06.405.205.200
    Colitis;C06.405.205.265
        Colitis, Ischemic;C06.405.205.265.115
        Colitis, Microscopic;C06.405.205.265.173
            Colitis, Collagenous;C06.405.205.265.173.500
            Colitis, Lymphocytic;C06.405.205.265.173.750
        Colitis, Ulcerative;C06.405.205.265.231
```

Fig. 4.2 Sample from the mtrees2010.txt file

In Fig. 4.1, it is presented as reduced representation of two descriptors: the useful information being contained in the *DescriptorUI and DescriptorName*, *TreeNumber* xml nodes:

In Fig. 4.2, it is presented as sample from the mtrees2010.txt file.

The hierarchical structure of each category can be established based on the tree number. For example, *Colitis* having the associated tree number *C06.405.20.265* has the following childs: *Colitis, Ischemic (C06.405.205.265.115)*, *Colitis, Microscopic (C06.405.205.265.173)*, *Colitis, Ulcerative (C06.405.205.265.231)*, etc. This observation will be taken into account when establishing the hierarchical relationships between concepts.

4.6 Mapping MeSH Content to the Ontology and Graphical Representation

The mapping of MeSH content to the ontology is made in an original manner during several steps and using the options presented in Fig. 4.3.

1. *Reducing the content of desc2010.xml file*—the size of this file is 276 MB. For our ontology, not all the information contained in this file is needed, and because of this, we have filtered the information, keeping only the XML nodes that are considered useful. The list of XML nodes contained in the reduced XML file is *DescriptorRecordSet*, *DescriptorRecord*, *DescriptorUI*, *DescriptorName*, *String*, *TreeNumberList*, *TreeNumber*, *ConceptList*, *Concept*, *TermList*, and *Term*. The application is receiving the path to the desc2010.xml file and the path for the reduced XML file (the location where it should be stored). After the *Start* button is pressed, the reduced file is generated having a size of 64 MB.

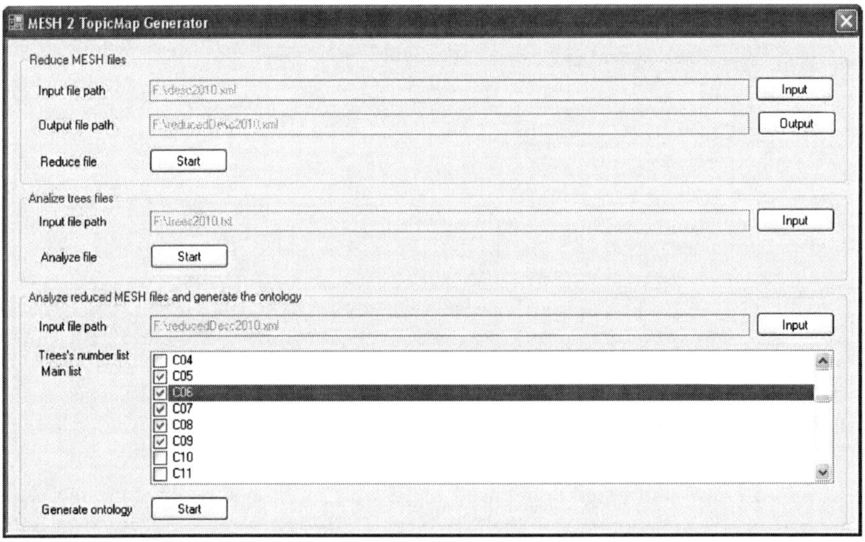

Fig. 4.3 Importing MeSH's content

2. *Analyzing the content of the mtrees2010.txt file*—this file is processed line by line. Each line is splitted using ";" as a separator. In this way, the name of the tree node and the tree number are identified. After all lines are processed, each tree number is used to identify its child nodes. The content of this file is used to detect the existing hierarchical relationships.
3. *Analyzing the content of the reduced XML file*—after specifying the path to the reduced file, this is automatically processed, and the information associated to each descriptor is extracted. It is possible to select the top-level categories. For example, if the user is selecting *C06* which represents *Digestive System Diseases*, then only the descriptors contained in this tree will be selected. This option is very useful for obtaining only the information needed for a specific purpose, for example, to have available only a list of concepts for annotating images belonging to the digestive diseases. At the end of this step, the list of descriptors and the list of related (associative) relationships are obtained. As it was mentioned, a descriptor may be related to another one. For example, a descriptor representing a specific disease may be related to another descriptor that represents a disease caused by that specific disease. Each descriptor will be represented as a concept in the ontology that will be created, and each relationship (hierarchical, associative) will represent a relationship having a specific type.

The ontology is represented as a Topic Map [28] using the XTM syntax [29]. In a Topic Map, a concept is represented by a *topic*, and a relationship is represented as an *association*. Table 4.1 presents the mapping of two descriptors (parent with **D003092** as *DescriptorUI* and **C06.405.205.265 and C06.405.469.158.188** as tree numbers **and** child with **D003093** as *DescriptorUI* and **C06.405.205.265.231**, **C06.405.205.731.249**, **C06.405.469.158.188.231**, and **C06.405.469.432.249** as tree numbers) to two topic items and the mapping of the hierarchical relationship between them to an association.

The Topic Map contains:

- Topics—each descriptor is mapped to a topic item having as unique identifier as the content of the DescriptorUI XML node. The base name of the topic is retrieved from the DescriptorName XML node. The tree node of this topic in the hierarchical structure of the Topic Map is established using the tree identifiers existing in the TreeNumber XML nodes. Usually, a MeSH descriptor can appear in multiple trees.
- Associations defined between topics—our ontology contains two types of associations:
  - Hierarchical—generated using the hierarchical structure of the MeSH trees and the tree identifiers defined for each concept (used to identify the concepts implied in the association).
  - Related to—a descriptor can be related to other descriptors. This information is mentioned in the descriptor content by a list of DescriptorUI values. In practice, a disease can be caused by other diseases.

Table 4.1 An example of mapping MeSH content to the ontology

Descriptor	Topic
<DescriptorRecord DescriptorClass = "1">	<topic id = “D003092”>
<DescriptorUI> D003092</DescriptorUI>	<instanceOf>
<DescriptorName>	<topicRef xlink:href="#concept"/>
<String>Colitis</String>	
</DescriptorName>	</instanceOf>
<TreeNumberList>	<baseName>
<TreeNumber> C06.405.205.265</TreeNumber>	<baseNameString> Colitis </baseNameString>
<TreeNumber>C06.405.469.158.188</TreeNumber>	</baseName>
</TreeNumberList>	</topic>
</DescriptorRecord>	
<DescriptorRecord DescriptorClass = "1">	<topic id = “D003093”>
<DescriptorUI> D003093 </DescriptorUI>	<instanceOf>
<DescriptorName>	<topicRef xlink:href="#concept"/>
<String>Colitis, Ulcerative </String>	
</DescriptorName>	</instanceOf>
<TreeNumberList> <TreeNumber>C06.405.205.265.231</TreeNumber>	<baseName>
<TreeNumber>C06.405.205.731.249</TreeNumber>	<baseNameString>Colitis, Ulcerative
<TreeNumber>C0C06.405.469.158.188.231</TreeNumber>	</baseNameString> </baseName>
<TreeNumber>C06.405.469.432.249</TreeNumber>	</topic>
</TreeNumberList>	
</DescriptorRecord>	
Association	
<association id=” D003092- D003093”>	
<instanceOf><topicRef xlink:href="#hierarchical"/></instanceOf>	
<member>	
<roleSpec><topicRef xlink:href="#parent"/></roleSpec>	
<topicRef xlink:href="# D003092"/>	
</member>	
<member>	
<roleSpec><topicRef xlink:href="#child"/></roleSpec>	
<topicRef xlink:href="# D003093 "/>	
</member>	
</association>	

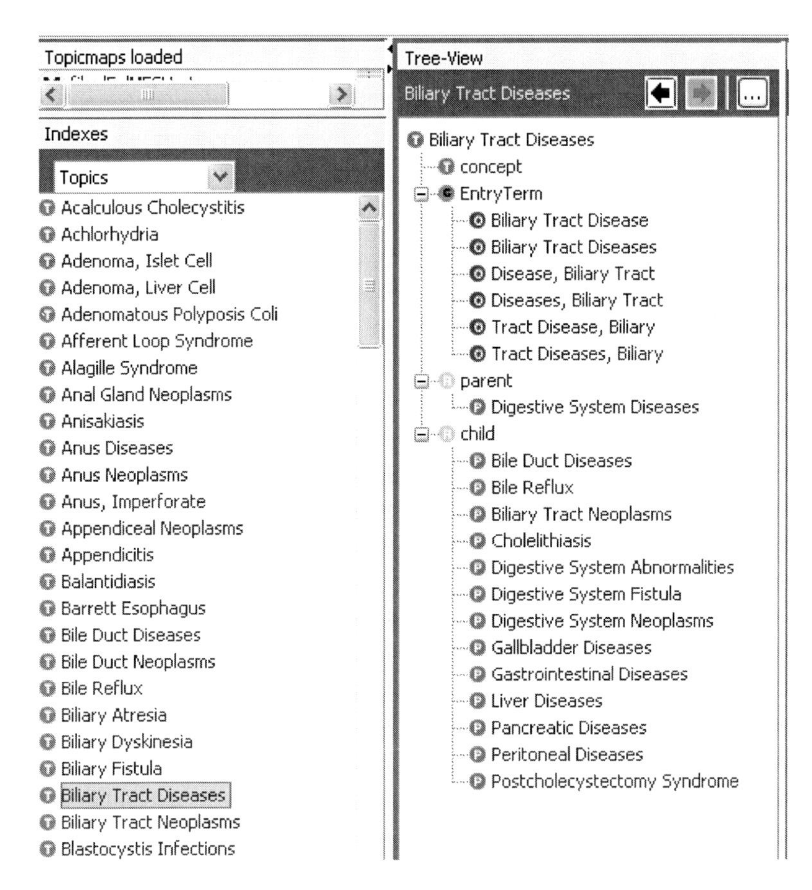

Fig. 4.4 List view and Tree view provided by TMNav

After the ontology is generated and represented as a Topic Map, it can be explored using the TMNav [38] software. TMNav is a Java application for browsing Topic Maps. The application can connect to and browse Topic Maps from any of the supported TM4J back ends. The navigation is presented in both a standard Swing GUI and a dynamic graph GUI using the TouchGraph library. The goal of the TMNav project is to create a framework for developing Topic Map browsing and editing applications and a reference implementation of a Topic Map editor. TMNav provides three views:

1. A *List view* containing a drop-down list that can be used for filtering; the user can select the option *Topics*, and after that the list containing all topics will be shown; other possible options are *Associations*, *Topic Types*, *Association Types, and Member Types*. This view can be seen in the left part of Fig. 4.4.
2. A *Tree view* containing details about a selected topic or association item. This view can be seen in the right part of Fig. 4.4.
3. A *Graph view* containing details about a selected topic or association item. This view can be seen in Fig. 4.5.

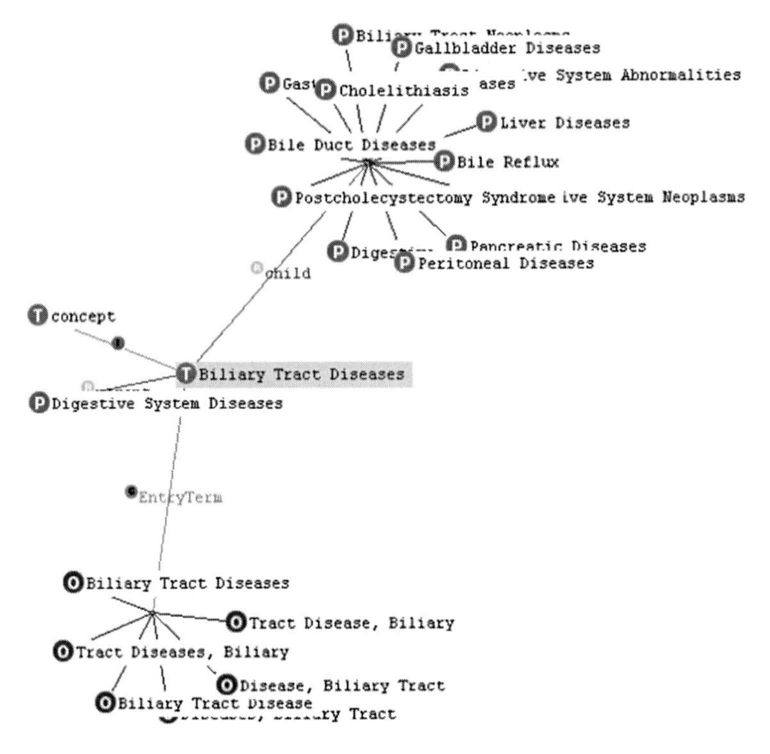

Fig. 4.5 Graph view provided by TMNav

An ontology can have a big size, and because of this a software that provides browsing capabilities needs to be used. By using a graphical representation of an ontology, it is offered an intuitive solution to a user that is not familiar with the details related to the syntax used to represent the concepts and the relationships within the ontology. Topic Maps are very powerful in their ability to organize information, but they may be very large. Intuitive visual user interfaces may significantly reduce users' cognitive load when working with these complex structures. Visualization is a promising technique for both enhancing users' perceptions of structure in large information spaces and providing navigation facilities. It also enables people to use natural tools of observation and processing—their eyes as well as their brains—to extract knowledge more efficiently and to find insights.

References

1. Moriya N, Hasharon R Ontology. The specification of a shared conceptualization, A review document source. http://www.iqlue.com/prosearch/ProSearchOntology.jsp?type=CMP. Accessed 26 Aug 2011
2. Staab S, Studer R (eds) (2009) Handbook on ontologies, 2nd edn. Series: International handbooks on information systems, Springer, Heidelberg
3. Gruber TR (1993) A translation approach to portable ontology specifications. Knowl Acquis 5:199–220
4. Noy NF, McGuinness DL (2001) Ontology development 101: a guide to creating your first ontology, Stanford University, Stanford. http://www-ksl.stanford.edu/people/dlm/papers/ontology101/ontology101-noy-mcguinness.html
5. The Generalized Upper Model. http://www.fb10.uni-bremen.de/anglistik/langpro/webspace/jb/gum/index.htm. Accessed 26 Aug 2011
6. Sensus ontology. http://www.isi.edu/natural-language/projects/ONTOLOGIES.html. Accessed 21 Aug 2011
7. Penman Upper Model. http://www.fb10.uni-bremen.de/anglistik/langpro/kpml/um89/um89-root.htm. Accessed 26 Aug 2011
8. Van Der P, Vet EP, Speel P, Mars NJI (1994) The Plinius ontology of ceramic materials. Workshop notes ECAI'94 workshop comparison of implemented ontologies: 187–205
9. Frame ontology. http://www-ksl.stanford.edu/knowledge-sharing/ontologies/html/frame-ontology/index.html. Accessed 21 Aug 2011
10. Thomas RG (1993) Toward principles for the design of ontologies used for knowledge sharing. In: Guarino N, Poli R (eds) Formal ontology in conceptual analysis and knowledge representation. Kluwer Academic, Deventer
11. Uschold M, Gruninger M (1996) Ontologies: principles, methods and applications. Knowl Eng Rev 11(2):93–137
12. Gennari J, Musen MA, Fergerson RW, Grosso WE, Crubezy M, Eriksson H, Noy NF, Tu SW (2003) The evolution of Protégé: an environment for knowledge-based systems development. Int J Hum Comp Stud 58(1):89–123
13. Knublauch H, Fergerson RW, Noy NF, Musen MA (2004) The Protégé OWL plugin: an open development environment for semantic web applications. In: 3rd international semantic web conference, Hiroshima, 2004
14. Web Ontology Language (OWL). http://www.w3.org/TR/owl-features/. Accessed 10 Aug 2011
15. Resource Description Framework (RDF). http://en.wikipedia.org/wiki/Resource_Description_Framework. Accessed 10 Aug 2011
16. DIG Interface. http://dig.sourceforge.net/. Accessed 10 Aug 2011
17. RacerPro. http://www.racer-systems.com/. Accessed 10 Aug 2011
18. FaCT++. http://owl.cs.manchester.ac.uk/fact++/. Accessed 10 Aug 2011
19. KAON2. http://kaon2.semanticweb.org/. Accessed 10 Aug 2011
20. Jena. http://jena.sourceforge.net/. Accessed 15 July 2011
21. Kalyanpur A, Parsia B, Sirin E, Cuenca-Grau B, Hendler J (2005) SWOOP, a web ontology editing browser. J Web Semantics 4(2):144–153
22. Rector AL, Rogers JE, Zanstra PE, Van Der Haring E. OpenGALEN: open source medical terminology and tools. In: Proceedings of the AMIA Symposium, Washington DC, 2003, p 982
23. Gangemi A, Pisanelli DM, Geri S (1999) An overview of the ONIONS project: applying ontologies to the integration of medical terminologies. Data Knowl Eng 31:183–220
24. http://lhncbc.nlm.nih.gov/cgsb_site/servlet/Turbine/template/research%2Cmedterm%2COntology.vm. Accessed 15 July 2011
25. The Gene Ontology Consortium (2000) Gene ontology: tool for the unification of biology. Nat Genet 25:25–29

26. The Gene Ontology Consortium (2001) Creating the gene ontology resource: design and implementation. Genome Res 11(8):1425–1433
27. Rosse C, Mejino JLV (2003) A reference ontology for bioinformatics: the foundational model of anatomy. J Biomed Inform 36:478–500
28. Topic Maps. http://www.topicmaps.org/. Accessed 15 July 2011
29. XTM syntax. http://www.topicmaps.org/xtm/. Accessed 20 July 2011
30. LTM. http://www.ontopia.net/download/ltm.html. Accessed 20 July 2011
31. AsTMa. http://astma.it.bond.edu.au/. Accessed 20 July 2011
32. Omigator. http://www.ontopia.net/solutions/omnigator.html. Accessed 20 July 2011
33. Empolis K42. http://notendur.hi.is/joner/eaps/cs_empo.htm. Accessed 20 July 2011
34. TM4L. http://compsci.wssu.edu/iis/nsdl/. Accessed 29 Aug 2011
35. Nelson SJ, Johnston D, Humphreys BL (2001) Relationships in medical subject headings. In: Bean CA, Green R (eds) Relationships in the organization of knowledge. Kluwer, Dordrecht, pp 171–184
36. http://www.nlm.nih.gov/mesh/2010/mesh_browser/MeSHtree.html. Accessed 20 Aug 2011
37. http://www.nlm.nih.gov/mesh/filelist.html. Accessed 20 Aug 2011
38. TMNav. http://tm4j.org/tmnav.html. Accessed 20 Aug 2011

Chapter 5
Medical Images Annotation

5.1 General Overview

Automatic image annotation is the process of assigning meaningful words to an image taking into account its content. This process is of great interest as it allows indexing, retrieving, and understanding of large collections of image data. There are two reasons that are making the image annotation a difficult task: the semantic gap, being hard to extract semantically meaningful entities using just low-level image features, and the lack of correspondence between the keywords and image regions in the training data. Image annotation has been a research topic of great interest for more than a decade, and several interesting techniques have been proposed. Most of these techniques define a parametric or nonparametric model to capture the relationship between image features and keywords. Each model has tried to improve the performance or to eliminate the limitations of a previous model. According to [1], the existing image annotation methods can be seen from supervised/unsupervised learning perspective.

Image annotation methods based on unsupervised learning consider keywords as textual features and can be classified in two categories from parametric/nonparametric perspective:

(a) *Parametric models* defined by a training stage to estimate the model parameters.
    The first attempt of using textual features for the automatic image annotation process was made in [2]. A co-occurrence model to represent the relationship between keywords and visual features was proposed. The image regions from the training data were clustered into a number of region clusters. For each training image, its keywords were propagated to each region. The major drawback of this model is that it assumes that if some keywords are annotated to an image, they are propagated to each region in this image with equal probabilities. This model required a large number of training samples to

L. Stanescu et al., *Creating New Medical Ontologies for Image Annotation: A Case Study*, SpringerBriefs in Electrical and Computer Engineering,
DOI 10.1007/978-1-4614-1909-9_5,

estimate the correct probability. The conditional keyword distribution of each individual image region is aggregated to generate the conditional keywords distribution for a test image.

Images were described in [3] using a vocabulary of blobs. Image regions were obtained using the normalized-cuts segmentation algorithm. For each image region, 33 features such as color, texture, position, and shape information were computed. An image is represented as a bag of image regions obtained by image segmentation and performed vector quantization on each of these region features. The regions were clustered using the K-means clustering algorithm into 500 clusters called "blobs." It used the classical IBM statistical machine translation model [4] to make a translation from the set of blobs associated to an image to the set of keywords for that image. This model does not propagate the keywords of an image to each region with equal probability. The association probability of a textual keyword to a visual word is taken as a hidden variable and estimated by the expectation-maximization (EM) [5] algorithm. From this reason, the annotation model called translation model was a substantial improvement of the co-occurrence model.

An approach based on a hidden Markov model (HMM) [6] is proposed in [7]. Each textual keyword is represented by a hidden state that can generate visual features following a per-state probability distribution. The training process tries to find the best correspondence of image regions and textual keywords and to estimate the parameters for each state. The annotation process of a new image is equivalent to recovering the most likely hidden state of each image region. The HMM model assumes a transition process between different states which is not always supported by real data.

A method to model the joint distribution of textual features and visual features instead of modeling the conditional distribution of textual keywords based on visual features was proposed in [8]. Based on their method, the authors define a document as a combination of visual features and textual features. The joint distribution of textual features and visual features is modeled using a hierarchical factor. The model assumes that a document belongs to a cluster denoted by the leaf nodes in the tree hierarchy. Having a document and the cluster it belongs to, the document can be generated using the aspect nodes on the path from the root node to the leaf node based on the hierarchical structure.

To find a conditional relationship between image features and textual features, the correlation latent Dirichlet allocation was proposed [9]. The dependence of the textual words on the image regions are modeled explicitly. This model is estimated using expectation-maximization algorithm and assumes that a Dirichlet distribution can be used to generate a mixture of latent factors. The approach relies on a hierarchical mixture representation of keyword classes, leading to a method that has a computational efficiency on complex annotation tasks.

The joint distribution of the image features and the textual words was represented in [10] using a probabilistic semantic model. It is assumed that there are a number of hidden semantics in an image each semantic having a probability to generate the global visual feature and the textual words.

For a specific semantic, the generation of visual features and textual words are independent from each other.

The automatic image annotation task has been explored in [11] using latent semantic analysis (LSA) [12] and probabilistic latent semantic analysis (PLSA) [13]. LSA and PLSA essentially model the co-occurrence relationship between any words including the textual words and visual words. These methods do not focus on the co-occurrence relationship between textual words and visual words. Using these methods, a document of image and texts can be represented as a bag of words, which includes the visual words which are vector-quantized image regions and textual words. Then LSA and PLSA can be deployed to project a document into a latent semantic space. Annotating images is achieved by keywords propagation in the latent semantic space.

(b) *Nonparametric models* that do not need to estimate any model parameters in the training stage, but they do need the whole training data for annotating a new image.

Automatic image annotation problem was seen in [14] as cross-lingual information retrieval and has applied the cross-media relevance model (CMRM) to perform both image annotation and ranked retrieval. This model is finding the training images which are similar to the test image and propagate their annotations to the test image. It is assumed that regions in an image can be described using a small vocabulary of blobs. Blobs are generated from image features using clustering. Based on a training set of images with annotations and using probabilistic models, it is possible to predict the probability of generating a word given the blobs in an image. This model can be used to automatically annotate and retrieve images given a word as a query. CMRM is much more efficient in implementation than the abovementioned parametric models because it does not have a training stage to estimate model parameters. The experimental results have shown that the performance of this model on the same data set was considerably better than the models proposed in [2, 3]. A drawback of the CMRM model is that it vector-quantized the image regions into image blobs, and this can reduce discriminative capability of the whole model.

An improved model called continuous cross-media relevance model (CRM) was proposed in [15]. The proposed approach learns the semantic of images which allows to automatically annotate an image with keywords and to retrieve images based on text queries. CRM preserves the continuous feature vector of each region, and this offers more discriminative power. A formalism that models the generation of annotated images is used. It is assumed that every image is divided into regions, each described by a continuous-valued feature vector. Starting from a training set of images with annotations, a joint probabilistic model of image features and words which allows the prediction of the probability of generating a word given the image regions is computed. It allows deriving the probabilities in a natural way, directly associates continuous features with words, and does not require an intermediate clustering stage The experiments have shown that the annotation performance of this continuous relevance model is substantially better than any other model tested on the same data set. It is almost an order of magnitude better (in terms of mean precision) than a model based on word-blob co-occurrence model, more than two and a half times better than a state of the art model derived from machine translation and 1.6 times as good as a discrete version of the relevance model.

A further extension of the CRM model called multiple Bernoulli relevance model (MBRM) was proposed in [16]. It was considered that the assumption of a multinomial distribution of keywords in CRM and CMRM favors prominent concepts in the images and equal length of annotation for each image. Because of this, they proposed to model the keyword distribution of an image annotation as a multiple Bernoulli distribution, which only represents the existence/nonexistence binary status of each word. The model assumes that a training set of images or videos along with keyword annotations is provided. Multiple keywords are provided for an image, and the specific correspondence between a keyword and an image is not provided. Each image is partitioned into a set of rectangular regions, and a real-valued feature vector is computed over these regions. The word probabilities are estimated using a multiple Bernoulli model and the image feature probabilities using a nonparametric kernel density estimate. The model is then used to annotate images in a test set. Their experimental results have shown that MBMR outperforms CMRM and CRM for the annotation of video frames.

Because the methods mentioned above predicted each word independently for a given test image and only the correlation between keywords and visual features was modeled, a coherent language model was proposed [17]. This model is extended from CMRM to model the correlation between two textual words. The model defines a language model as a multinomial distribution of words. It takes into account the word-to-word correlation by estimating a coherent language model for an image. Instead of estimating the conditional distribution of a single word, the conditional distribution of the language model is estimated. The correlation between words can be explained by a constraint on the multinomial distribution that the summation of the individual words distribution is equal to one. The prediction of one word has an effect on the prediction of another word. This new approach has two important advantages: it is able to automatically determine the annotation length to improve the accuracy of retrieval results, and it can be used with active learning to significantly reduce the required number of annotated image examples.

Automatic image annotation can be also performed using graph-based methods. Such an example is GCap [18]. An image is represented as a set of regions each of which being described by a visual feature vector. The whole training data is used to construct a graph that has three types of node: *image node* representing an image, *region node* representing an image region, and *word node* representing a textual keyword. For a test image, the image regions are obtained by unsupervised image segmentation. An image node representing the test image and several region nodes representing the image regions in the test image are added to the graph constructed on the training set. The annotation process is modeled as a random walk with restarts (RWR) [19] on the graph.

An adaptive graph model [20] constructed on the training data was proposed for image annotation. The graph has only one type of node, the image node. Each image node is connected to its k-nearest neighbors. The number of nearest neighbors connected to each image node, k, is different to each other and decided by an adaptive process. The annotation probability of each word to the images is represented in a ranking order matrix. For a new image, the ranking order matrix is computed by iteratively updating the matrix by the manifold ranking algorithm [21].

Image annotation methods based on *supervised learning* are considering keywords as different class labels. Using this approach, the process for annotating an image with a keyword becomes similar with the classification of that image to a particular class. Existing approaches to image annotation based on image classification fall into three categories:

1. *Global scene-oriented classification methods*—extract a global feature descriptor from an image and then use a statistical classifier for image classification.
   A real-time ALIPR image search engine [22] is using multiresolution 2D hidden Markov models to model concepts determined by a training set. Categorized images are used to train a dictionary of hundreds of statistical models each representing a concept. Images of any given concept are regarded as instances of a stochastic process that characterizes the concept. To measure the extent of association between an image and the textual description of a concept, the likelihood of the occurrence of the image based on the characterizing stochastic process is computed. A high likelihood indicates a strong association.

   Quantitative spatial and photometric relationships [23] were incorporated within and across regions in low-resolution images for natural scene image classification. The discriminative capability of different visual features for "city" vs. "landscape" scene classification was examined in [24], and it was demonstrated that the edge direction-based features have the best discriminative capability on their data set.

   Support vector machines (SVM) [25] were used in [26] to solve the general image classification problem. The semantics of a scene image was decomposed into two levels [27]: the primitive semantics at the patch level and the scene semantics at the image level. The learning of primitive semantics is based on a supervised clustering of the patch features.

   A method for hierarchical classification of vocational images was proposed in [28]. At the highest level, images are classified as indoor or outdoor. The probability density of each scene class is modeled using vector quantization [29]. Using global multiscale orientation features, it was possible to classify "city"/ "suburb" images [30].

   In [31], an image annotation framework based on hierarchical mixture modeling of the probability density estimation of each class was proposed. Each image is represented as a set of patch features, and the distribution of these patch features for each concept is modeled as a Gaussian mixture model. All concepts are modeled by a hierarchical Gaussian mixture model (Hier-GMM).

The occurring frequency of different concepts in an image was used in [32] as the intermediate features for scene image classification.

A soft categorization method of images based on the Bayes point machines (BPM) [33] was proposed in [34]. A Bayesian hierarchical model extended from latent Dirichlet allocation (LDA) was proposed in [35] to learn natural scene categories.

A good performance in scene classification was obtained in [36] by combining probabilistic latent semantic analysis (PLSA) [13] and a KNN classifier.

Spatial pyramid matching for scene image classification was applied in [37] by partitioning an image into increasingly fine subregions and taking each subregion as a bag of visual words.

2. *Local object-oriented classification methods*—classify images by object names. The image content assigned to the labels is usually a part of the image. Some examples of these class labels include "balloon," "water," and "people." An image can be broken down into a bag of regions, and in this way, the image annotation can be formulated as a multiple instance learning (MIL) problem [38]. In the MIL setting, the object to be classified is a bag of instances instead of a single instance.

   The first attempt for applying MIL techniques to natural scene image classification was made in [39]. A distinction between terms such as "sky," "waterfall," and "mountain" was made. Each image was represented as a bag of subimages of 2×2 pixels. The training of this MIL is made through maximizing the diverse density.

   An asymmetric support vector machine method (ASVM) [40] was proposed to solve the MIL problem and have applied it to region-based image annotation. This method is called ASVM-MIL and extends the conventional support vector machines to the MIL setting by introducing asymmetrical loss functions for false positive and false negatives. The training algorithm can be formulated as a standard quadratic programming problem which is very efficient.

3. *Multilevel classification methods*—assign class labels in a hierarchical structure including both scene-oriented class and object-oriented class.
   Global scene-oriented classification and the local object-oriented classification approaches are advantageous for handling certain types of image categories. There are some cases when it is needed to annotate images that contain both global scene-oriented class and local object-oriented class elements. For this reason, a comprehensive approach that can annotate these two types of class together is needed.

   Multilevel image annotating has been performed in [41–43]. In [43], keywords into different level of semantics are organized in a hierarchical structure. At the lowest level are those concepts which can be represented by salient objects. The individual detectors of these salient objects are trained separately.

In [44] for building the concept ontology, a semisupervised algorithm to learn it from the LabelMe data set [45] and from WordNet was proposed [46]. In [47], the current methods for extracting semantic information from images are classified in two main categories from text/image-based perspective:

(a) *Text-based methods*—the system analyzes the text associated with the image objects and extracts those that appear to be relevant. Text-based methods use additional knowledge about images that exist in associated text, ontologies, and can be divided into three main categories:

Ontology-based methods—these methods utilize an ontology that exists in the form of lists of keywords, hierarchical categories, or lexicographic databases. Ontology offers the possibility to characterize a given domain by conceptualizing and specifying knowledge in terms of entities, attributes, and relationships. The usage of specialized ontologies in medicine, art, and history in order to perform domain-specific annotations has been presented in [48, 49].

Context-based methods—images may exist in the context of a multimedia document, and such contextual content can be utilized to annotate images. Context-based examples of automatic Web-based image annotation and retrieval systems include search engines such as Google image search. The engine analyzes the text on the Web page adjacent to an image, its caption, and other factors in order to determine the image content. The weight chainNet model [50] is one of the representative works for Web image annotation and retrieval.

Human-based methods—these methods assist humans to assign annotations by providing convenient user interfaces. Human-based methods are utilized for images without associated text (i.e., there is minimal or no usable context). Intelligent user interfaces are provided in order to minimize the manual operation and to provide a few initial options for users to choose from. The Aria system that can be used by the users to create annotations for images when editing e-mail messages is presented in [51].

(b) *Image-based methods*—rely on extracting semantic information directly from image content [47]. An image-based method is composed of two steps. In the first step, one or more models between content features and keywords are derived by using a set of previously annotated images. In the second step, the models are used to annotate new images and/or regions. Image-based annotation methods can be classified in two types:

Regional feature–based methods—most image annotation methods rely on regional features. Image segmentation and/or partitioning techniques are used to detect objects in an image. After this step, the completed models are generated by calculating the probability of co-occurrence of words with regional image features. The models are used to annotate new images. Starting from a training set of annotated images, regional feature–based methods attempt to discover the statistical links between visual features and words followed by estimating the correlations between words and regional image features. Starting from a training set of images T, one or more of the following steps are performed:

- *Segmentation*—segmentation algorithms like Blobworld [52] or normalized cuts [53] are used to divide images into regions, followed by the extraction and quantification of features from the regions. Regions are described by a set of low-level features like color, texture, shape, etc.
- *Clustering*—regions are clustered into a set of similar regions called a blob. Each region is represented by high-dimensional features. The assumption made is that similar regions belong to the same cluster. The annotation performance is influenced strongly by the quality of clustering. Clustering algorithms such as K-means [54] assume that all features are equally important.
- *Correlation*—the last step is to analyze the correlation between words and regions in order to discover hidden semantics. This can be the most difficult task, since image data sets usually do not provide explicit correspondence between the two.

The regional feature–based methods can be classified further as:

- *Word-region mapping*. The word-region process maps frequent words to every region but is very difficult to find such learning data. To handle this problem, multiple instance learning (MIL) [38] can be used. To learn a concept, MIL uses a set of bags labeled positive or negative. Alternatively, it can be used expectation maximization (EM) [5] which is an iterative optimization method for finding maximum likelihood estimates of unknown parameters in probabilistic models. co-occurrence model [2] and machine translation model [3] are two existing word-region mapping models.
- *Word-image mapping*. Assigning words to image regions can cause many errors due to the oversegmentation of images. Word-image mapping uses regional features to map frequent words to every image. Three existing word-image mapping statistical models are using this approach: hierarchical aspect model [8], the cross-media relevance model [14], and the two-dimensional multiresolution hidden Markov model (2D MHMM) [55].

Global feature–based methods—they make use of global image features and are very attractive when creating a low-cost framework for feature extraction and image classification. The tradeoff compared to regional feature–based methods is that global features typically do not capture detailed information about individual objects. For this reason, some types of annotations may not be possible using global-based features. Two recent examples of the global feature annotation process are: content-based soft annotation (CBSA) [34] and SVM-based annotation [56].

5.2 Annotation Systems in the Medical Domain

Some annotation systems used in the medical domain are presented below.

I2Cnet (image indexing by content network) [57] provides services for content-based management of images in healthcare. I2Cnetmedical image annotation service allows specialists to annotate groups of images, communicate them to any user by e-mail, and search for medical images and annotations based on image content and annotation. An I2Cnet annotation contains a number of parts: details which specify regions of interest in a graphical manner, notation text which is a textual field linked to a detail, overlays that group together multiple details and notation texts, annotation message, and the pointers of the annotation. Each annotation is associated with a property object that contains metadata like the annotation author, subject, relevant keywords, etc. I2Cnet is organized as a network of I2Cnet servers, which interoperate with Image Management and Communication Systems (IMACS) and offer services related to the content-based management of images.

Hierarchical medical image annotation system presented in [58] uses support vector machines (SVM)-based approaches. The system is evaluating the combination of three different methods. Global image descriptors are concatenated with an interest points' bag of words to build a feature vector. An initial annotation of the data is performed using two known methods and disregarding the hierarchy of theIRMA code. The hierarchy is taken into consideration by classifying consecutively its instances. At the end, pair-wise majority voting is applied between these methods by simply summing strings in order to produce a final annotation.

Oxalis [59] represents a distributed image annotation architecture allowing the annotation of an image with diagnoses and pathologies. Oxalis enables a user to display a digital image, to annotate the image with diagnoses and pathologies using a free-form drawing tool, to group images for comparison, and to assign images and groups to schematic templates for clarity. Images and annotations are stored in a central database where they can be accessed by multiple users simultaneously. The design of Oxalis enables developers to modify existing system components or add new ones, such as display capabilities for a new image format, without editing or recompiling the entire system. System components can be notified when data records are created, modified, or removed and can access the most current system data at any point. Even if Oxalis was designed for ophthalmic images, it represents a generic architecture for image annotation applications.

SENTIENT-MD (Semantic Annotation and Inference for Medical Knowledge Discovery) is a new-generation medical knowledge annotation and acquisition system [60]. The system allows a precise semantic annotation of medical knowledge in natural language text. For this, the approach is to semantically annotate natural language parse trees that are transformed into annotated semantic networks for inferring general knowledge from text. The system is used in nuclear cardiology.

An Ontology Annotation Tree browser (*OAT*) [61] was created to represent, condense, filter, and summarize the knowledge associated with a list of genes or proteins. Because ontologies are a good way to represent knowledge, this novel interactive annotation browser incorporates two ontologies: one ontology of medical subject headings (MeSH) and gene ontology (GO), for an improved interpretation of gene lists.

Volume-object annotation system (*VANO*) is a cross-platform image annotation system enabling the visualization and the annotation of 3D volume objects including nuclei and cells [62]. VANO can be used to create masks and annotations for objects from scratch, to correct the segmentation of an existing mask, or to enter, edit, or correct the annotation of the set of objects in the current mask. The combination of a spreadsheet that lists all objects and pop-ups for individual objects in an image view makes it easy to survey annotation and keep track of hundreds of objects. The image files are stored in TIFF format, and the annotation is stored in simple CSV (comma separated values) format, so it can easily be parsed and used by other programs.

CMAS (Collaborative Medical Annotation System) [63] system was created in order to allow medical professionals to easily annotate digital medical records that contain medical images or videos. The CMAS system uses an innovative video annotation technology called Active Shadows that captures a virtual presence interacting with a displayed image and overlays on top of a digital image. With Active Shadows, the expert opinion and presence (a doctor, a patient) is combined with the information inside the images. Active Shadows immerses the viewer in an image or video and simultaneously captures the viewer's experience. The CMAS system structures the annotation of digital medical records such that image/video annotations from multiple sources, at different times, and from different locations can be maintained within a historical context.

ImageCLEF [64–67] was one of the first campaigns that organized evaluation events for image retrieval applications. ImageCLEF began as a pilot experiment in 2003 with a bilingual ad hoc retrieval task using a database of images with accompanying texts in one language.

In 2005, a medical image annotation task was added to ImageCLEF, and participation increased strongly, especially for the newly offered task. In 2006, the medical annotation task was continued with an enlarged data set and a higher number of classes, and the database used for medical retrieval grew to approximately 50,000 images. In 2007, the medical annotation task was extended toward hierarchical classification; the medical retrieval database grew to approximately 70,000 images.

The automatic medical image annotation has evolved from a simple classification task with about 60 classes to a task with almost 120 classes. From the beginning, it was clear that the number of classes cannot be scaled indefinitely and that the number of classes that are desirable to be recognized in medical applications is far too big. To solve this problem, a hierarchical class structure such as the image retrieval in medical applications (IRMA) code can be a solution because it supports the creation of a set of classifiers for subproblems. The classes in the years 2005 and 2006 were based on the IRMA code. They were created by grouping similar codes in a single class.

In 2007, the task has changed, and the objective is to predict complete IRMA codes instead of simple classes. In 2007, the medical annotation process was based on the previous one; 1,000 new images were added and used as test data. The training and the test data of 2006 were used as training and development data, respectively.

5.3 Cross-Media Relevance Model Based on an Object-Oriented Approach

For the annotation process of the medical images, we have created an extension of the cross-media relevance model (CMRM) model-based of an object-oriented approach in order to achieve greater flexibility. CMRM model was chosen as an annotation model because it was proved that it can produce better annotation results than other existing models. This model offers the possibility to perform semantic-based image retrieval, providing a ranked list of images for a given query.

5.3.1 Cross-Media Relevance Model Description

CMRM [14] is a nonparametric model for image annotation and assigns words to the entire image. It is assumed that image regions can be described using a small vocabulary of blobs. In this context, a blob represents a cluster of image regions. The set of blobs are obtained by applying clustering techniques (e.g., K-means algorithm) on image features. Each blob is assigned a unique integer to serve as its identifier. Having available a training set of images with annotations and using a probabilistic-based approach, the probability of generating a word given the blobs in an image is calculated. Given a new test image, it can be segmented into regions, and region features can be computed. The blob which is closest to it in cluster space is assigned to it. The model is using some principles defined for the relevance-based language models [68, 69]. These models were used to perform query expansion in a more formal manner being used for ad hoc retrieval and cross-language retrieval.

CMRM can be used in two ways:

1. Document-based expansion—the blobs corresponding to each test image are used to generate words and associated probabilities from the joint distribution of blobs and words. Each test image is annotated with a vector of probabilities for all the words in the vocabulary.
2. *Query expansion*—the query word(s) is used to generate a set of blob probabilities from the joint distribution of blobs and words. This vector of blob probabilities is compared with the vector of blobs for each test image using Kullback-Leibler (KL) divergence, and the resulting KL distance is used to rank the images.

Table 5.1 Explanation of the elements used in the equations

Item	Description
$P(w \mid J)$, $P(w \mid J)$	Probabilities of selecting the word w, the blob b from the model of the image J
$\#(w, J)$	Actual number of times the word w occurs in the caption of image J
$\#(w, T)$	Is the total number of times w occurs in all captions in the training set T
#(b, J)	Reflects the actual number of times some region of the image J is labeled with blob b
$\#(b, T)$	Is the cumulative number of occurrences of blob b in the training set
$\lvert J \rvert$	Stands for the count of all words and blobs occurring in image J
$\lvert T \rvert$	Denotes the total size of the training set
$P(J)$	Prior probabilities are be kept uniform over all images in T being estimated with Eq. 5.5
α and β	Smoothing parameters were used as: $\alpha = 0.1$ and $\beta = 0.9$

According to this model, a test image I is annotated by estimating the joint probability of a keyword w and a set of blobs [14]:

$$P(w, b_1, \ldots, b_m) \sum_{J \in T} P(J) P(w, b_1, \ldots, b_m \,|J) \tag{5.1}$$

For the annotation process, the following assumptions are made:

(a) A collection C of unannotated images is given.
(b) Each image I from C to can be represented by a discrete set of blobs $I = \{b_1 \ldots b_m\}$
(c) There exists a training collection T, of annotated images, where each image J from T has a dual representation in terms of both words and blobs: $J = \{b_1 \ldots b_m;\ w_1 \ldots w_n\}$
(d) $P(J)$ is kept uniform over all images in T.
(e) The number of blobs and words in each image (m and n) may be different from image to image.
(f) No underlying one to one correspondence is assumed between the set of blobs and the set of words; it is assumed that the set of blobs is related to the set of words.

Based on a generative language modeling approach, it is assumed that for each image I there exists some underlying probability distribution $(P.|I)$. This distribution is seen as the relevance model of I. It is assumed that the observed image representation $(b_1, \ldots, b_m)$ is the result of m random samples from $(P.|I)$.

$P(w, b_1, \ldots, b_m|J)$ represents the joint probability of keyword w and the set of blobs $(b_1, \ldots, b_m)$ conditioned on training image J. In CMRM, it is assumed that, given image J, the events of observing a particular keyword w and any of the blobs $(b_1, \ldots, b_m)$ are mutually independent. This means that $P(b_1, \ldots, b_m|J)$ can be written as [14] (Table 5.1):

$$P(w, b_1, \ldots, b_m|J) = P(w|J) \prod_{(i=1)}^{m} P(b_i|J) \tag{5.2}$$

$$P(w|J) = (1 - \alpha_J)\frac{\#(w,J)}{|J|} + \alpha_J\frac{\#(w,T)}{|T|}. \tag{5.3}$$

$$P(b|J) = (1 - \beta_J)\frac{\#(b,J)}{|J|} + \beta_J\frac{\#(b,T)}{|T|}. \tag{5.4}$$

$$P(J) = \frac{1}{|T|}. \tag{5.5}$$

5.3.2 *The Database Model*

The database used to store the information needed for the annotation process is an open-source object-oriented database called db4o [70] having bindings to both the. NET and Java platforms. We have chosen this approach because an object-oriented model offers support for storing complex objects as sets, lists, trees, or other advanced data structures. It is very easy to use db4o because it is native to Java and.NET, and the data objects are stored exactly in the way they are defined by the application. It is not required anymore to predefine or maintain a separate, rigid data model, because the model is now created and updated by db4o itself during a transaction. Unlike string-based query languages, db4o offers truly native and object-oriented data access APIs like language integrated queries for querying the database, query by example which makes it easy to search for matching object, retrieval by object graph allowing to use normal methods to retrieve objects on demand without creating new queries. The elimination of data transformation in db4o leads to less demand on CPU or persistence operations, which shifts critical resources to the application logic and query processing [71].

For db4o, the following methods are available for querying objects:

(a) *Query by Example* (*QBE*)—a query expression is based on template objects being fast and simple to implement. This method is an optimal solution for simple queries that are not using logical operators. The matching objects are returned by the query in a set, namely, an instance of the IObjectSet type [72].

(b) *Simple Object Data Access* (*SODA*)—a query expression is based on query graphs. This method builds a query graph by navigating references in classes and imposing constraints. SODA has several disadvantages because a query is expressed as a set of method calls that explicitly define the graph, and it is not similar in any way to traditional querying techniques. Another important disadvantage is the fact that attribute names are strings; therefore SODA queries are not type-safe.

(c) *Native Queries* (*NQ*)—this querying approach express the query in a.NET or Java—compliant language by writing a method that returns a Boolean value. The method is applied to all objects stored and the list of matching object instances is returned. db4o will attempt to optimize native query expressions and execute them against indexes and without instantiating actual objects, where this is possible.

(d) *Language Integrated Query* (*LINQ*)—is the recommended db4o querying interface for.NET platforms. db4o querying syntax has got even easier with the introduction of.NET LINQ queries. LINQ allows you to write compile-checked db4o queries, which can be automatically updated when a field name changes and which are supported by code autocompletion tools.

db4o offers support for client/server interactions, each interaction being one of the following three types:

(a) *Networking*—is the traditional way of operating in most database solutions. Remote clients open a TCP/IP connection to send/retrieve data to/from the db4o server.
(b) *Embedded*—the client and the server are run on the same machine. The communication between the server and the client is the same as in networking mode, but the work is entirely made within one process. A db4o server is opened on port 0 for a database file thereby declaring that no networking will take place.
(c) *Out-of-band signaling*—the information sent does not belong to the db4o protocol and does not consist of data objects but, instead, is completely user-defined. This mode uses a message passing communication interface.

5.3.3 The Annotation Process

The annotation process based on the object-oriented approach contains the following steps for each new image:

1. *Image segmentation*—using our original segmentation algorithm presented in a previous chapter, a method called *SegmentImage* generates a list of image regions. At the end of the segmentation process, each region will be represented as a *Region* object. The following statement reflects this process:

   List < Region > regions = SegmentImage (imagePath)

2. *Features extraction*—from each region, a feature vector being represented by a *FeaturesVector object is extracted.* This object is set as a property for the corresponding region object. At the end of this process performed by a method called *ExtractFeatures,* a list of FeaturesVector objects is obtained. The following statement reflects this process:

   List < FeaturesVector > features = ExtractFeatures
   (List < Region > regions)

3. *Identifying the Blob object corresponding to a Region object*—in our implementation, a *Blob* object (representing a cluster of regions) contains an *AverageFeaturesVector* object obtained by making an average of all *FeaturesVector* objects belonging to the regions assigned to that blob. In order to identify the *Blob* object

that should be assigned to a *Region* object, the Euclidian distance between the components of the *AverageFeaturesVector* object belonging to a *Blob* object and the components of the *FeaturesVector* object belonging to that region is computed. The *Blob* object for which the minimum distance is obtained will be assigned to the *Region* object. This process is performed using a method called *IdentifyBlob* having the following implementation:

```
Public Blob IdentifyBlob (Region r) {
  -- db is the object used to access the database called Database.yap
 IObjectContainer db =Db4oFactory.OpenFile("Database.yap");
 -- using LINQ to obtain a list of ComputedDistance objects
IEnumerable<ComputedDistance> distances=from Blob blob in db
       select newComputedDistance {
   Distance = ComputeDistance(blob.AverageFeaturesVector, r.FeaturesVector),
   BlobItem = blob;
       }
-- sorting ascending the list and selecting the first value
   ComputedDistance min = distances.OrderBy(pd => pd.Distance).First();
-- assigning the Blob object to the Region object
      r.Blob = min.BlobItem ;
      return r.Blob;
  }
```

4. *Representing the image as a discrete set of blobs identifiers*—for the annotation process, we need also the list of distinct *Blob* objects assigned to the current image. For the object-oriented approach, this list can be computed using the following method based on LINQ and applying the *IdentifyBlob* method for each region:

```
Public List<Blob> DetectBlobs (List<Region> regions) {
  List<Blob> distinctBlobs = new List<Blob>();
  Blob minBlob;
  foreach (Region region in regions){
    minBlob = IdentifyBlob (region);
 -- add the Blob object in the list if not already added
     if (!distinctBlobs.Contains(min.BlobItem)){
       distinctBlobs.Add(min.BlobItem); }
     }
     return distinctBlobs;
    }
```

5. *Estimating the joint probability of each Word object w*—based on the set of *Blob* objects detected above, the joint probability described by the equation (1) is estimated. This probability for a *Word* object w can be made using the method called *PWBs* (presented in Table 5.2) having as main input parameters the *Word* w, the set of *Blob* objects detected above, and the list of *Image* objects from the training set.

6. *Annotating the image*—after calculating the probability of each *Word* object w, a list containing these values is obtained. The list is sorted in a descending order to have the words considered to be more relevant for the analyzed image on top positions. Based on the length of the annotation (the number of words to be used for annotation), a number of *n Word* objects to represent the annotation of the analyzed image are selected.

The process described using previous steps is implemented by the *AnnotateImage* method having the following implementation:

```
Public List<Word> AnnotateImage (string imagePath, int n) {
-- Obtaining the list of all Word and Blob objects from the database
 IEnumerable<Word> words = from Word w in db select w;
 IEnumerable<Blob> allBlobs = from Blob b in db select b;
-- Obtaining the list of all Image objects from the training set T existing in the database
 IEnumerable<Image> T  = from Image img in db select img;
-- Equivalent to |T|
 int cardT = words.Count() + allBlobs.Count();
-- The list of Region objects detected at step 1
 List<Region> regions = SegmentImage (imagePath);
-- The list of distinct Blob objects detected at step 2
 List<Blob> blobs = DetectBlobs(regions);
-- This list will contain the probabilities computed for each Word object
 List<Probability> probabilities = new List<Probability>();
 double value;
 foreach (Word w in words){
 -- Calculating the probability for the Word w
   value = PWBs(w, blobs, T,db, cardT);
 -- Creating a new Probability object
   Probability p = new Probability();
 p.Word = w;
 p.Value = value;
 probabilities.Add(p);
}
-- The list of probabilities is sorted in a descending order based on the Value field
 probabilities = probabilities.OrderByDescending(pd => pd.Value).ToList();
 List<Word> annotationWords = probabilities.GetFirstWords(n);
}
```

The annotation process is summarized in Fig. 5.1.

The mapping used between the CMRM model and the object-oriented approach is presented in Table 5.2, and the classes used for the annotation process are presented in Table 5.3.

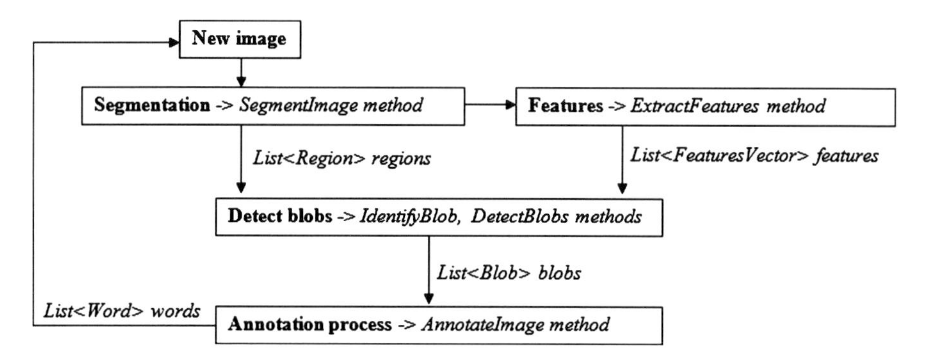

Fig. 5.1 Annotation process diagram

Table 5.2 The mapping used for the object-oriented approach

CMRM model	Object-oriented model
$P(w\|J)$	Public double PWJ(Word w, Image J, IObjectContainer db, int cardT)
$P(b\|J)$	Public double PBJ(Blob b, Image J, IObjectContainer db, int cardT)
$P(w, b_1, \ldots, b_m\|J)$	Public double PWBsJ(Word w, List < Blob > blobs, Image J, IObjectContainer db, int cardT)
$P(w, b_1, \ldots, b_m)$	Public double PWBs(Word w, List < Blob > blobs, List < Image > T, IObjectContainer db, int cardT)
$P(Q\|J)$	Public double PQJ(List < Word > query, Image J, IObjectContainer db, int cardT)
$P(b\|Q)$	Public double PBQ(Blob b, List < Word > query, IObjectContainer db, int cardT)
$-KL(Q\|\|J)$	Public double KLQJ(List < Word > query, Image J, IObjectContainer db, int cardT)

Table 5.3 The classes used by the annotation model

Classes	Members	Member's type
Image	PictureName	String
	Regions	List < Region>
Region	Index	Int
	AssignedBlob	Blob
	AssignedWord	Word
	FeaturesVectorItem	FeaturesVector
	MatrixFilePath	String
Blob	Index	Int
	AverageFeaturesVector	FeaturesVector
FeaturesVector	Features	List < double>
Word	Name	String
	OriginalIndex	Int
HierarchicalRelationship	ParentWord	Word
	ChildWord	Word
	Index	Int

5.3.4 Measures for the Evaluation of the Annotation Task

Evaluation measures [47] are considered to evaluate the annotation performance of an algorithm. Let T' represent a test set, $J \in T'$ be a test image, W_J be its manual annotation set, and W_J^a be its automatic annotation set. The performance can be analyzed from two perspectives:

1. *Annotation perspective*. Two standard measures that are used for analyzing the performance from the annotation perspective are:

   (a) *Accuracy*. The accuracy of the autoannotated test images is measured as the percentage of correctly annotated words, and for a given test image, $J \subset T'$ is defined as [47]:

$$accuracy = \frac{r}{|W_J|} \tag{5.6}$$

   Where variable r represents the number of correctly predicted words in J. The disadvantage of this measure is represented by the fact that it does not take into account for the number of wrong-predicted words with respect to the vocabulary size $|W|$.

   (b) *Normalized score* (*NS*). It is extended directly from accuracy and penalizes the wrong predictions. This measure is defined as [47]:

$$\text{NS} = \frac{r}{|W_J|} - \frac{r'}{|W| - |W_J|} \tag{5.7}$$

   Where variable r' denotes the number of wrong predicted words in J.

2. *Retrieval perspective*. Retrieval performance measures can be used to evaluate the annotation quality. Autoannotated test images are retrieved using keywords from the vocabulary. The relevance of the retrieved images is verified by evaluating it against the manual annotations of the images. Precision and recall values are computed for every word in the test set. Precision is represented by the percentage of retrieved images that are relevant. Recall is represented by the percentage of relevant images that are retrieved. For a given query word wq, precision and recall are defined as [47]:

$$precision(w_q) = \frac{|\{J \in T' | w_q \in W_J^a \wedge w_q \in W_J\}|}{|\{J \in T' | w_q \in W_J^a\}|} \tag{5.8}$$

$$recall(w_q) = \frac{|\{J \in T' | w_q \in W_J^a \wedge w_q \in W_J\}|}{|\{J \in T' | w_q \in W_J\}|} \tag{5.9}$$

Table 5.4 An example of automatic annotation

Index	Diagnostic	R	WJ	Accuracy
0	Esophagitis	2	4	2/4 = 0.5
1	Peptic ulcer	3	4	3/4 = 0.75
2	Rectocolitis	2	3	2/3 = 0.66
3	Colitis	1	3	1/3 = 0.33
4	Duodenal ulcer	2	4	2/5 = 0.5
5	Gastritis atrophic	1	4	1/4 = 0.25
6	Gastritis hypertrophic	1	3	1/3 = 0.33
7	Stomach ulcer	3	4	3/4 = 0.75
8	Gastric varices	1	3	1/3 = 0.33
9	Peptic ulcer perforation	2	4	2/4 = 0.5

The average precision and recall over different single-word queries are used to measure the overall quality of automatically generated annotations. The precision and recall can be combined into a single measure called the $F1$-measure being defined as [47]:

$$F1(w_q) = \frac{2 * precision(w_q) * recall(w_q)}{precision(w_q) + recall(w_q)} \tag{5.10}$$

It can be useful to measure the number of single-word queries for which at least one relevant image can be retrieved using the automatic annotations. This metric compliments average precision and recall by providing information about how wide the range of words that contribute to the average precision and recall is. It is defined as [47]:

$$|\{w_q | precision(w_q) > 0 \wedge recall(w_q) > 0\}| \tag{5.11}$$

5.3.5 *Experimental Results*

In order to evaluate the annotation performance, we have used a testing set of 400 images that were manually annotated and not included in the training set used for the CMRM model. Each image had one of the diagnostics mentioned in Table 5.4. This set was then automatically annotated using the CMRM model. The performance of the annotation process was analyzed from the two perspective presented above:

(a) *Annotation Perspective*
 The number of relevant words automatically assigned was compared against the number of relevant words manually assigned by computing an accuracy value. Using this approach for each test image, we have obtained an evaluation having

Table 5.5 Statistical evaluation from precision-recall perspective

Index	Word	Precision	Recall
0	Esophagitis	0.31	0.34
1	Peptic ulcer	0.25	0.32
2	Rectocolitis	0.41	0.52
3	Colitis	0.45	0.41
4	Duodenal ulcer	0.28	0.38
5	Gastritis atrophic	0.32	0.54
6	Gastritis hypertrophic	0.12	0.49
7	Stomach ulcer	0.30	0.18
8	Gastric varices	0.37	0.42
9	Peptic ulcer perforation	0.44	0.32
		Mean precision	Mean recall
		0.32	0.39

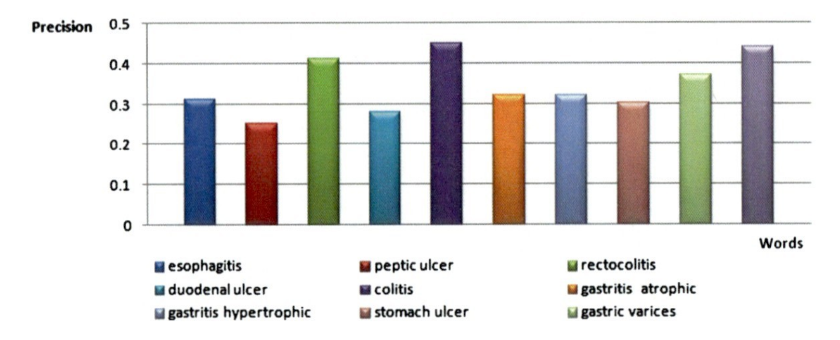

Fig. 5.2 Precision chart

the structure presented as in Table 5.4. For each diagnostic, we have included in this table, presented as example, only one value of the accuracy.

R represents the number of relevant words automatically assigned, and WJ represents words manually assigned. After computing the accuracy value for each image, a medium accuracy value equal to 0.47 was obtained.

(b) *Retrieval Perspective*

After each image from the testing set is autoannotated, a list of distinct words (used for annotating these images) is computed. Let us suppose that the list contains k words, $\{w_1 \ldots w_k\}$. For each word, the relevance of the images from the test set and containing that word in their annotation is verified. This is easily done by looking at the manual annotations of each image. Precision and recall values are calculated for each word. At the end of this process, a mean precision and recall values are computed. The statistical evaluation that was obtained is presented in Table 5.5 and in a graphical manner in Figs. 5.2 and 5.3.

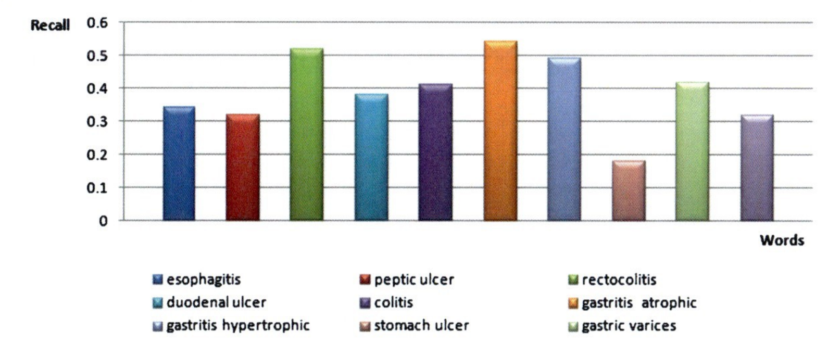

Fig. 5.3 Recall chart

5.4 Conclusions

In this chapter, we have presented an overview of the existing methods for image annotation and a detailed description of an original object-oriented extension of the CMRM model. All steps required by the annotation process have been clearly identified and presented in an intuitive manner. There are several studies that are treating the image annotation process, but there is no clear presentation of the steps that should be applied.

Because object-oriented databases expose means through which objects can be queried and stored using the same model that it employed by the application's programming language, we have decided to use db4o. db4o is a powerful and simple to use database that can be integrated easier into an application. Using this database, a greater flexibility and extensibility was obtained.

The performance of the annotation process has been evaluated from the annotation and retrieval perspectives. The mean values obtained for precision (0.32) and recall (0.39) are very similar with the ones (mean precision 0.33, mean recall 0.37) obtained in [14] for the CMRM model with fixed annotation. Even if the experiments were performed for a data set that was different from the one used in [14], it can be concluded that our object-oriented extension produces good results.

Future work will involve an extension of the data set in order to have more pictures for the existing diagnostics that are currently treated in our approach and for new ones. We believe that this extension will improve the performance and the evaluation of the model. Other improvements can be achieved by using a better feature extraction or by using continuous features.

References

1. Wang Y (2008) Automatic image annotation and categorization, PhD thesis, University of London, September
2. Mori Y, Takahashi H, Oka R (1999) Image-to-word transformation based on dividing and vector quantizing images with words. In: MISRM'99 first international workshop on multimedia intelligent storage and retrieval management, Orlando, 1999

3. Duygulu P, Barnard K, de Freitas N, Forsyth D (2002) Object recognition as machine translation: learning a lexicon for a fixed image vocabulary. In: Seventh European conference on computer vision, Copenhagen, 2002, pp 97–112
4. Brown P, Pietra SD, Pietra VD, Mercer R (1993) The mathematics of statistical machine translation: parameter estimation. Comput Linguist 19(2):263–311
5. Dempster AP, Laird NM, Rubin DB (1977) Maximum likelihood from incomplete data via the em algorithm. J R Stat Soc Ser B (Methodological) 39(1):1–38
6. Lawrence RR (1989) A tutorial on hidden Markov models and selected applications in speech recognition. Proc IEEE 77(2):257–286
7. Arnab G, Pavel I, Sanjeev K (2005) Hidden Markov models for automatic annotation and content-based retrieval of images and video. In: Proceedings of ACM SIGIR international conference on research and development in information retrieval (SIGIR), Salvador, 2005, pp 544–551
8. Barnard K, Forsyth DA (2001) Learning the semantics of words and pictures. In: Proceedings of IEEE international conference on computer vision (ICCV), Vancouver, 2001, pp 408–415
9. Blei DM, Jordan MI (2003) Modeling annotated data. In: Proceedings of ACM SIGIR international conference on research and development in information retrieval (SIGIR), Toronto, 2003, pp 127–134
10. Zhang R, Zhang Z(M.), Li M, Ma WY, Zhang HJ (2005) A probabilistic semantic model for image annotation and multi-modal image retrieval. In: Proceedings of IEEE international conference on computer vision (ICCV), Beijing, 2005, pp 846–851
11. Monay F, Gatica-Perez D (2004) PlSA-based image auto-annotation: constraining the latent space. In: Proceedings of ACM international conference on multimedia (ACM MULTIMEDIA), New York, 2004, pp 348–351
12. Deerwester SC, Dumais ST, Landauer TK, Furnas GW, Harshman RA (1990) Indexing by latent semantic analysis. J Soc Inform Sci 41(6):391–407
13. Hofmann T (2001) Unsupervised learning by probabilistic latent semantic analysis. Mach Learn 42(1–2):177–196
14. Jeon J, Lavrenko V, Manmatha R (2003) Automatic image annotation and retrieval using cross-media relevance models. In: Proceedings of ACM SIGIR international conference on research and development in information retrieval (SIGIR), Toronto, 2003, pp 119–126
15. Lavrenko V, Manmatha R, Jeon J (2004) A model for learning the semantics of pictures. In: Proceedings of advances in neural information processing systems (NIPS), Vancouver, 2004
16. Feng SL et al. (2004) Multiple bernoulli relevance models for image and video annotation. In: Proceedings of IEEE conference on computer vision and pattern recognition (CVPR), Washington, DC, 2004, pp 1242–1245
17. Jin R, Chai JY, Si L (2004) Effective automatic image annotation via a coherent language model and active learning. In: Proceedings of ACM international conference on multimedia (ACM MULTIMEDIA), New York, 2004, pp 892–899
18. Pan JY, Yang HJ, Faloutsos C (2004) Duygulu P GCap: graph-based automatic image captioning. In: Proceedings of IEEE international conference on computer vision and pattern recognition workshop, Washington, DC, 2004, pp 146–149
19. Tong H, Faloutsos C, Pan JY (2006) Fast random walk with restart and its applications. In: Proceedings of the international conference on data mining, Hong Kong, 2006, pp 613–622
20. Liu J, Li M, Ma WY, Liu Q, Lu H (2006) An adaptive graph model for automatic image annotation. In: Proceedings of the ACM SIGMM international workshop on multimedia information retrieval (MIR), Santa Barbara, 2006, pp 873–877
21. Zhou D, Weston J, Gretton A, Bousquet O, Scholkopf B (2004) Ranking on data manifolds. In: Proceedings of advances in neural information processing systems (NIPS), Vancouver and Whistler, 2004
22. Li J, Wang J (2003) Automatic linguistic indexing of pictures by a statistical modeling approach. IEEE Trans Pattern Anal Mach Intell 25:1075–1088

23. Lipson P, Grimson E, Sinha P (1997) Configuration based scene classification and image indexing. In: Proceedings of the 1997 conference on computer vision and pattern recognition, San Juan, 1997, pp 1007–1010
24. Vailaya A, Jain A, Zhang HJ (1998) On image classification: city images vs. landscapes. Pattern Recognit 31(12):1921–1935
25. Cristianini N, Shawe-Taylor J (2000) An introduction to support vector machines and other kernel-based learning methods. Cambridge University Press, New York
26. Chapelle O, Haffner P, Vapnik V (1999) Support vector machines for histogram-based image classification. IEEE Trans Neural Netw 10(5):1055–1064
27. Yiu Fung C, Fock Loe K (1999) Learning primitive and scene semantics of images for classification and retrieval. In: Proceedings of ACM international conference on multimedia (ACM MULTIMEDIA), Orlando, 1999, pp 9–12
28. Vailaya A, Figueiredo M, Jain A, Zhang H (2001) Image classification for content-based indexing. IEEE Trans Image Process 10(1):117–130
29. Gray R (1986) Vector quantization. IEEE Signal Process Mag 1(2):4–29
30. Gorkani MM, Picard RW (1994) Texture orientation for sorting photos "at a glance". In: Proceedings of IEEE international conference in pattern recognition, Jerusalem, 1994, pp 459–464
31. Carneiro G, Vasconcelos N (2005) Formulating semantic image annotation as a supervised learning problem. In: Proceedings of IEEE conference on computer vision and pattern recognition (CVPR), San Diego, 2005, pp 163–168
32. Vogel J, Schiele B (2007) Semantic modeling of natural scenes for content-based image retrieval. Int J Comput Vis (IJCV) 72(2):133–157
33. Herbrich R, Graepel T, Campbell C (2001) Bayes point machines. J Mach Learn Res (JMLR) 1:245–279
34. Chang EY, Goh K, Sychay G, Wu G (2003) CBSA: content-based soft annotation for multimodal image retrieval using Bayes point machines. IEEE Trans Circuits Syst Video Technol (CSVT) 13(1):26–38
35. Fei-Fei L, Perona P (2005) A Bayesian hierarchical model for learning natural scene categories. In: Proceedings of IEEE conference on computer vision and pattern recognition (CVPR), San Diego, 2005, pp 523–525
36. Bosch A, Zisserman A, Munoz X (2006) Scene classification via PLSA. In: Proceedings of European conference on computer vision (ECCV), Graz, 2006, pp 1134–1137
37. Lazebnik S, Schmid C, Ponce J (2006) Beyond bags of features: spatial pyramid matching for recognizing natural scene categories. In: Proceedings of IEEE conference on computer vision and pattern recognition (CVPR), New York, 2006, pp 988–991
38. Dietterich TG, Lathrop RH, Lozano-Perez T (1997) Solving the multiple-instance problem with axis-parallel rectangles. Artif Intell 89(1–2):31–71
39. Maron O, Ratan AL (1998) Multiple-instance learning for natural scene classification. In: Proceedings of IEEE international conference on machine learning (ICML), Madison, 1998, pp 341–349
40. Yang C, Dong M, Hua J (2006) Region-based image annotation using asymmetrical support vector machine-based multiple-instance learning. In: Proceedings of IEEE conference on computer vision and pattern recognition (CVPR), New York, 2006, pp 1057–1063
41. Fan J, Gao Y, Luo H (2004) Multi-level annotation of natural scenes using dominant image components and semantic concepts. In: Proceedings of ACM international conference on multimedia (ACM MULTIMEDIA), New York, 2004, pp 540–547
42. Fan J, Gao Y, Luo H, Xu G (2004) Automatic image annotation by using concept-sensitive salient objects for image content representation. In: Proceedings of ACM SIGIR international conference on research and development in information retrieval (SIGIR), Sheffield, 2004, pp 361–368
43. Gao Y, Fan J (2006) Incorporating concept ontology to enable probabilistic concept reasoning for multi-level image annotation. In: Proceedings of the ACM SIGMM international workshop on multimedia information retrieval (MIR), Santa Barbara, 2006, pp 79–88

44. Gao Y, Fan J, Xue X, Jain R (2006) Automatic image annotation by incorporating feature hierarchy and boosting to scale up SVM classifiers. In: Proceedings of ACM international conference on multimedia (ACM MULTIMEDIA), Santa Barbara, 2006, pp 901–910
45. Russell BC, Torralba A, Murphy KP, Freeman WT (2005) LabelMe: a database and web-based tool for image annotation. Technical report, Massachusetts Institute of Technology, MIT AI Lab Memo AIM-2005–025
46. Miller GA (1992) WordNet: a lexical database for English. In: Proceedings of the workshop on speech and natural language, San Mateo, 1992, pp 483–483
47. Shah B, Benton R, Wu Z, Raghavan V (2007) Chapter VI: Automatic and semi-automatic techniques for image annotation. In: Zhang Y-J (ed) Semantic-based visual information retrieval. IRM Press, Hershey
48. Hu B, Dasmahapatra S, Lewis P, Shadbolt N (2003) Ontology-based medical image annotation with description logics. In: Proceedings of the IEEE conference on tools with artificial intelligence, Sacramento, 2003, p 77
49. Soo V, Lee C, Li C, Chen S, Chen C (2003) Automatic semantic annotation and retrieval based on sharable ontology and case-based learning techniques. In: Proceedings of the joint conference on digital libraries, Houston, 2003, pp 61–72
50. Shen H, Ooi B, Tan K (2000) Giving meanings to WWW images. In: Proceedings of the ACM conference on multimedia, Marina del Rey, 2000, pp 39–47
51. Lieberman H, Rosenzweig E, Singh P (2001) Aria: an agent for annotating and retrieving images. IEEE Comput 34(7):57–61
52. Carson C, Thomas M, Belongie S, Hellerstein J, Malik J (1999) Blobworld: a system for region-based image indexing and retrieval. In: Proceedings of the conference on visual information systems, Amsterdam, 1999, pp 509–516
53. Shi J, Malik J (2000) Normalized cuts and image segmentation. IEEE Trans Pattern Anal Mach Intell 22(8):888–905
54. Hartigan J, Wong M (1979) A K-means clustering algorithm. Appl Stat 28(1):100–108
55. Li J, Gray R, Olshen RA (2000) Multiresolution image classification by hierarchical modeling with two dimensional hidden Markov models. IEEE Trans Inform Theory 34(5):1826–1841
56. Feng H, Shi R, Chua T (2004) A bootstrapping framework for annotating and retrieving WWW images. In: Proceedings of the ACM conference on multimedia, New York, 2004, pp 960–967
57. Catherine EC, Xenophon Z, Stelios CO (1997) I2Cnet medical image annotation service. Med Inform 22(4):337–347 (Special Issue)
58. Igor FA, Filipe C, Joaquim F, Pinto da C, Jaime SC (2010) Hierarchical medical image annotation using SVM-based approaches. In: Proceedings of the 10th IEEE international conference on information technology and applications in biomedicine, Korfu, 2010
59. Daniel E (2003) OXALIS: a distributed, extensible ophthalmic image annotation system, Master of Science Thesis. University of Pittsburgh
60. Baoli L, Ernest VG, Ashwin R (2007) Semantic annotation and inference for medical knowledge discovery. In: NSF symposium on next generation of data mining (NGDM-07), Baltimore, 2007
61. Bresell A, Servenius Bo, Persson B (2006) Ontology annotation Treebrowser: an interactive tool where the complementarity of medical subject headings and gene ontology improves the interpretation of gene lists. Appl Bioinformatics 5(4):225–236
62. Peng H, Long F, Myers EW (2009) VANO: a volume-object image annotation system. Bioinformatics 25(5):695–697
63. Lin I-J, Chao H (2006) CMAS, a rich media annotation system for medical imaging. Prog Biomed Opt Imaging 7(31):614506.1–614506.8
64. ImageCLEF. http://www.imageclef.org/. Accessed 25 Aug 2011
65. Hersh W, Kalpathy-Cramer J, Jensen J (2006) Medical image retrieval and automated annotation: OHSU at ImageCLEF. In: CLEF, Alicante, 2006, vol 4730, pp 660–669
66. Gospodnetic O, Hatcher E (2005) Lucene in action. Manning Publications, Greenwich

67. Nabney IT (2004) Netlab: algorithms for pattern recognition. Springer, London
68. Lavrenko V, Croft W (2001) Relevance-based language models. In: Proceedings of the 24th annual international ACM SIGIR conference, New Orleans, 2001, pp 120–127
69. Lavrenko V, Choquette M, Croft W (2002) Cross-lingual relevance models. In: Proceedings of the 25th annual international ACM SIGIR conference, Tampere, 2002, pp 175–182
70. db4objects. http://www.db4o.com/. Accessed 25 Aug 2011
71. Db4o Developer Community. http://developer.db4o.com/. Accessed 25 Aug 2011
72. Paterson J, Edlich S, Hoerning H, Hoerning R (2006) The definitive guide to db4o. Apress, New York

Chapter 6
Semantic-Based Image Retrieval

6.1 General Overview

Visual information has become an important factor in all aspects of our society. The large visual data make the dynamic research to focus on the problem of how efficiently to capture, store, access, process, represent, describe, query, search, and retrieve their contents. Research on semantic-based image retrieval is concerned on topics like human knowledge and behavior, distributed indexing and retrieval, indexing and retrieval for large databases, information mining for indexing, machine-learning approaches, higher-level interpretation, human-computer interaction, object classification and annotation, object recognition and scene understanding, relevance feedback and association feedback, semantic modeling for retrieval, and semantic representation and description [1]. The existing semantic gap between semantic meaning and the perceptual feeling has gained an important attention. Smeulders et al. [2] defined the semantic gap as "the lack of coincidence between the information that one can extract from the visual data and the interpretation that the same data have for a user in a given situation." Retrieval based on semantic meaning tries to extract the cognitive concept of a human by combining the low-level features in some way. Semantic meaning extraction based on feature vectors is difficult because feature vectors indeed cannot capture the perception of human beings [3].

The semantic image retrieval methods have been categorized roughly into the following classes [4]:

(a) Automatic scene classification in whole images by statistically based techniques
(b) Methods for learning and propagating labels assigned by human users
(c) Automatic object classification using knowledge-based or statistical techniques
(d) Retrieval methods with relevance feedback during a retrieval session

A semantic multimedia retrieval system consists of two components [5]. The first component links low-level physical attributes of multimedia data to high-level

L. Stanescu et al., *Creating New Medical Ontologies for Image Annotation: A Case Study*, SpringerBriefs in Electrical and Computer Engineering,
DOI 10.1007/978-1-4614-1909-9_6,

semantic class labels. The second component is represented by domain knowledge or any information that makes the system more capable to handle the semantics of the query.

Semantic retrieval requires the use of a cognitive model. This can be a feature element construction model [6] that tries to enhance the view-based model while importing some useful inferences from image-based theory. A feature element is the discrete unit extracted from low-level data that represent the distinct or discriminating visual characteristics that may be related to the essence of the objects. A novel cognitive model is proposed when trying to achieve the semantic retrieval. Two types of retrieval mode are available in the new system. Both types try to analysis the semantic concept in the query image or semantic command. The matching from the object to the feature element is carried out to obtain the final result.

According to [7], the semantic level is higher than the feature level, while the affective level is higher than the semantic level. Affection is associated with some abstract attributes that are quite subjective.

A knowledge-driven framework using ontologies as the means for knowledge representation is investigated in [8] for image semantic analysis and retrieval in the domain of outdoor photographs. In order to implement the framework for performing analysis and retrieval of visual content at a semantic level, two ontologies, analysis and domain, are defined and integrated appropriately. Both ontologies are expressed in RDF(S). The domain ontology formalizes the domain semantics, providing the conceptualization and vocabulary for the visual content annotations and the subsequent semantic retrieval. The analysis ontology is used to guide the analysis process and support the detection of certain concepts defined in the domain ontology. The main classes of the domain ontology account for the different types of objects and events depicted in an outdoor photograph. Relations are defined to model additional information regarding the person who took the photograph, the date the photograph was taken, and the corresponding location. The goal of knowledge-assisted semantic visual content analysis is to extract semantic descriptions from low-level image descriptions by exploiting prior knowledge about the domain under consideration. The developed analysis ontology can be seen as extending the initial domain ontology with qualitative and quantitative descriptions for those domain concepts that are to be detected automatically. In order to realize the ontology-based retrieval component, the semantic-enabled functionalities of an existing RDF knowledge base are exploited. Sesame [9] was selected for storing and querying the RDFS ontology and metadata. Concept-based queries are formulated by expanding the domain concepts hierarchy and by selecting the class or the classes that correspond to the content in which the user is interested. The resulting query is the conjunction of the selections made in the expanded ontology concept hierarchies.

A semantic learning method for content-based image retrieval using the analytic hierarchical process (AHP) has been proposed [10]. The AHP provides a good way to evaluate the fitness of a semantic description that is used to represent an image object. The idea behind this work is the problem of assigning semantic descriptions to the objects of an image that can be formulated as a multicriteria preference problem.

AHP is a powerful tool for solving multicriteria preference problems. In this approach, a semantic vector consisting of the fitness values of a given image semantics is used to represent the semantic content of the image according to a predefined concept hierarchy. The method for ranking retrieved images according to their similarity measurements integrates the high-level semantic distance and the low-level feature distance. Based on the semantic vectors, the database images are clustered. For each semantic cluster, the weightings of the low-level features (like color, shape, and texture) used to represent the content of the images are calculated by analyzing the homogeneity of the class. The values of weightings setting to the three low-level feature types are diverse in different semantic clusters for retrieval. The proposed semantic learning scheme provides a way to bridge the gap between the high-level semantic concept and the low-level features for content-based image retrieval. Experimental results showed that the performance of the proposed method is excellent when compared with text-based semantic retrieval techniques and content-based image retrieval methods.

Ontology-based frameworks for manual image annotation and semantic retrieval include the ones presented in [11, 12], considering photographs of animals and art images. In [11], the use of background knowledge contained in ontologies to index and search collections of photographs is explored. An annotation strategy and a tool for formulating annotations and searching for specific images is developed. Both ontologies (annotation, domain) are using general terminology.

In [12] is presented a tool for semantic annotation and search in a collection of art images. Multiple existing ontologies like Art and Architecture Thesaurus, WordNet, ULAN, and Iconclass are used to support this process. Knowledge-engineering aspects such as the annotation structure and links between the ontologies are taken into account. The tool provides two types of semantic search. With the first search option, the user can search for concepts at a random place in the image annotation. General concept search retrieves images that match the query in some part of the annotation. The second search option allows the user to exploit the annotation template for search purpose.

A new technique called cluster-based retrieval of images by unsupervised learning (CLUE) [13] exploits similarities among database images for improving user interaction with image retrieval systems. The major difference between a cluster-based image retrieval system and traditional CBIR systems lies in the two processing stages: selecting neighboring target images and image clustering. The two stages are the major components of CLUE. CLUE retrieves image clusters by applying a graph-theoretic clustering algorithm to a collection of images in the vicinity of the query. In CLUE, the clustering process is dynamic, and the clusters formed depend on the images that are retrieved in response to the query. CLUE attempts to capture semantic concepts by learning the way that images of the same semantics are similar and retrieving image clusters instead of a set of ordered images. CLUE is a general approach that can be combined with any real-valued symmetric similarity measure.

An ontology-based information extraction is proposed by the MUMIS (multi-media indexing and searching) project [14] to improve the results of information retrieval in multimedia archives through a domain-specific ontology, multilingual lexicons, and reasoning algorithms to integrate cross-modal content annotations. The domain-specific ontology, the multilingual lexicons, and the information passed between the different processing modules are encoded in XML. The content used as a test case is a collection of video recordings of soccer matches in three different languages: Dutch, English, and German. The link between the ontology and the three languages consists of a flexible XML format which maps concepts to lexical expressions. Every concept can have several children of the class term-lang. The annotations produced by the information extraction modules are first merged into one single annotation of knowledge about the soccer match. This approach improves the reliability of the search results.

A cascading framework for combining intra-image and interclass similarities in image retrieval motivated from probabilistic Bayesian principles has been proposed in [15]. Support vector machines [16] are employed to learn local view-based semantics based on just-in-time fusion of color and texture features. A new detection-driven, block-based segmentation algorithm is designed to extract semantic features from images. The detection-based indexes serve as input for support vector learning of image classifiers in order to generate class-relative indexes. During image retrieval, both intra-image and interclass similarities are combined to rank images. Experiments using Query by Example on 2,400 genuine heterogeneous consumer photos with 16 semantic queries showed that the combined matching approach is better than matching with single index.

In [17], the authors present the Imagea (image analogies) system that is using a novel application of the *Analogy-Making as Perception* model described in [18] in order to solve the content-based image retrieval task. This model uses a collection of independent agents to combine low-level perception of image features with high-level concepts. Two important aspects included in this model are represented by the automatic selection of an appropriate representation and the integration of this representation-building process with analogy-making. The Imagea system measures the similarity between two binary images by creating an analogy based on the objects in the images where objects are identified using strong segmentation. The system then applies features to these input objects, and these features are not included in the input. Imagea addresses the Representation Problem by integrating the mapping process with the representation-building process. When a new mapping between two images is built, the representation-building process begins searching for more instances of the features and relationships used in that mapping.

A two-stage retrieval process is described in [19]. Users perform queries by using a set of local semantic concepts and the size of the image area to be covered by the particular concept. In first stage, only small patches of the image are analyzed. In the second stage, the patch information is processed, and the relevant images are retrieved. In this two-stage retrieval system the precision and recall of retrieval can be modeled statistically. Based on the model, closed-form expressions that allow for the prediction as well as the optimization of the retrieval performance are designed. In the proposed retrieval system, users describe the images they are looking for by using a set of local semantic concepts (e.g., “sky,” “water,” “building,” “rocks,” etc.)

and the size of the image area to be covered by the particular concept. The technical realization of the retrieval is split into two stages. In the first stage, the database images are analyzed by these concept detectors. The detectors return a binary decision whether a particular image region contains the concept (positive patch) or not (negative patch). Each image is subdivided into a regular grid of patches, each comprising 1% of the image. The patch-wise information of the concept detectors is processed according to the user interval to actually retrieve a set of images. The performance optimization affects the selection of the appropriate concept detector in first stage and the setting of an internal parameter, the so-called system interval.

A new object categorization method for image retrieval is presented in [20]. This method is based on a visual concept ontology and involves machine-learning and knowledge representation techniques. The ontology contains several types of concepts (spatial concepts and relations, color concepts, and texture concepts). The proposed approach is designed for semantic interpretation of isolated objects of interest.

The method contains three phases:

(a) *Knowledge acquisition phase*—this phase is driven by a visual concept ontology. Knowledge acquisition process consists of achieving the following tasks: domain taxonomy acquisition, ontology-driven visual description of domain, and image sample management (annotation and manual segmentation of samples of object classes of interest). Sample annotation consists of labeling each manually segmented region of interest by a domain class name.
(b) *Learning phase*—the role of visual concept learning is to learn representative samples of visual concepts used during knowledge acquisition phase. Visual concept learning fills the gap between ontological concepts and image level. Visual concept learning consists of training a set of detectors to recognize visual concepts contained in the ontology. This learning is done using a set of training vectors computed during feature extraction on manually segmented and annotated regions of interest. The visual concept ontology is used because the learning process is done in a hierarchical way by using ontological tree structure. Visual concept learning is composed of three steps: training set building, feature selection, and training.
(c) *Categorization phase*—the categorization process is initiated by a categorization request which contains an image of the object to categorize. The object of interest has to be segmented from background. To achieve object extraction, a region growing segmentation algorithm is used. Initial seeds are placed at the corners of the image. Local matching is performed between current class attribute values and visual concepts recognized by the detectors trained during the learning process. Global matching consists of evaluating if current class matches the object to be recognized. This matching is done by combining probabilities computed during local matching.

A novel strategy that combines textual and visual clustering results to retrieve images using semantic keywords and autoannotate images based on similarity with existing keywords is proposed in [21]. It is assumed that images that fall in to the same text cluster can be described with common visual features of those images. Images are first clustered according to their text annotations using C3M (cover-coefficient-based clustering methodology) [22]. The images are also segmented into regions and then clustered based on low-level visual features using K-means clustering algorithm on the image regions. The feature vector of the images is then changed to a dimension equal to the number of visual clusters where each entry of the new feature vector signifies the contribution of the image to that visual cluster. A matrix is created for each textual cluster, where each row in the matrix is the new feature vector for the image in that textual cluster. A feature vector created for the query image is then appended to the matrix for each textual cluster. The images in the textual cluster that give the highest coupling coefficient are considered for retrieval. Annotations of the images in that textual cluster are considered as candidate annotations for the query image.

An image retrieval methodology suited for search in large collections of heterogeneous images is presented in [23]. The proposed approach employs a fully unsupervised segmentation algorithm to divide images into regions. An automatic mapping is performed between low-level features describing the color, position, size, and shape of the resulting regions and appropriate intermediate-level descriptors. Using this approach, a simple vocabulary termed object ontology is formed. The object ontology is used to allow the qualitative definition of the high-level concepts of the user queries in a human-centered fashion. During the querying process, irrelevant image regions are rejected using the intermediate-level descriptors. A relevance feedback mechanism employing the low-level features is invoked to produce the final query results.

A new relevance feedback technique is proposed in [24]. This technique uses the normal mixture model for the high-level similarity metric of the user's intention and estimates the unknown parameters from the user's feedback. The approach is based on a novel hybrid algorithm where the criterion for the selection of the display image set is evolved from the most informative to the most probable as the retrieval process progresses.

In [25], the authors proposed a combination of the semantic image retrieval model with text-based retrieval using a novel region-based inverted file indexing method. Images are translated into textual documents which are then indexed and retrieved the same way as the conventional text-based search. A different approach from existing semantic image retrieval methods is applied. First, it is created a semantic dictionary, and each image document is translated into a set of textual keywords. Then the image database is indexed using the inverted file so that image retrieval is done the same way as textual document retrieval. During the indexing process, the importance of each semantic keyword is determined based on the region size the keyword is associated to. The experimental results showed that this method provides text-based search efficiency and also a better performance than the conventional low-level image retrieval.

Automatic image annotation problem and its application to multimodal image retrieval is treated in [26]. The authors proposed a probabilistic semantic model in which the visual features and the textual words are connected via a hidden layer which constitutes the semantic concepts to be discovered to explicitly exploit the synergy among the modalities. The association of visual features and textual words is determined in a Bayesian framework such that the confidence of the association can be provided. In the proposed probabilistic model, a hidden concept layer which connects the visual feature and the word layer is discovered by fitting a generative model to the training image and annotation words through an expectation-maximization (EM)-based iterative learning procedure. The system supports both image-to-text (i.e., image annotation) and text-to-image retrievals.

IRMA (image retrieval in medical applications) [27] is a cooperative project of the Department of Diagnostic Radiology, the Department of Medical Informatics, Division of Medical Image Processing, and the Chair of Computer Science VI at the Aachen University of Technology (RWTH Aachen). The aim of the project is the development and implementation of high-level methods for content-based image retrieval with prototypical application to medico-diagnostic tasks on a radiologic image archive. It is intended to perform semantic and formalized queries on the medical image database which includes intra- and interindividual variance and diseases. The system classifies and registers radiologic images in a general way without restriction to a certain diagnostic problem or question. Methods of pattern recognition and structural analysis are used to describe the image content in a feature-based, formal, and generalized way.

The IRMA project goals are:

(a) *Automated classification* of radiographs based on global features with respect to imaging modality, direction, body region examined, and biological system under investigation.
(b) *Identification of image features* that are relevant for medical diagnosis. These features are derived from a priori classified and registered images. The database contains primary and secondary digitized radiographs, which have been classified by radiologists. Using local image analysis, a hierarchical Blob representation is obtained describing the image structure.

IRMA was implemented as a development environment, which allows the distributed storage of different resource types. Feature extraction algorithms can be executed within a network cluster. Resources are images, extracted features, as well as the feature extraction algorithms. Extracted features are stored within the database, and they are available for evaluation during queries, such as Query by Examples (QBE).

6.2 Semantic-Based Image Retrieval Using the Cross-Media Relevance Model

Generally speaking, for the image retrieval, task can be identified in two cases:

(a) *Text-based*—the user submits a textual query, and the system searches for images with similar keyword(s) in its captions.

(b) *Image-based*—the system tries to determine the most similar images to a given query image by using low-level visual features such as color, texture, or shape.

Recent approaches have proposed a semantic-based approach in order to assign a semantic meaning to the whole image or to its regions. This approach tries to determinate the strong relationships between keywords and types of visual features associated with images. The relationships are used to retrieve images based on a textual query. The association keyword/visual feature allows retrieving nonannotated but similar images to those retrieved by a classical textual query.

In the context of the cross-media relevance model (CMRM) [28], the task of semantic image retrieval takes into consideration a text query $Q = w_1...w_k$ and a collection C of images. The goal is to retrieve the images that contain objects described by the keywords or, more generally, rank the images I by the likelihood that they are relevant to the query. Text retrieval systems cannot be used because the images $I \in C$ are assumed to have no caption.

The cross-media relevance model allows two models for semantic-based image retrieval [28]:

(a) Given a query word, the first model called *probabilistic annotation-based cross-media relevance model* (*PACMRM*) can be used to rank the images using a language-modeling approach. This method is very useful for ranked retrieval.

Given a query $Q = w_1...w_k$ and the image $I = \{b_1...b_m\}$, the probability of drawing Q from the model of I is defined as [28]:

$$P(Q|I) = \prod_{j=1}^{k} P(w_j|I) \tag{6.1}$$

where $P(w_j|I)$ is computed using the Eqs. 5.1, 5.2, 5.3, and 5.4 of the CMRM model.

The probability of being relevant for the query Q is computed for each image. The list of probabilities is sorted in a descending order, and the first n images are considered to be most relevant.

(b) The second model corresponds to query expansion and is called *direct-retrieval cross-media relevance model* (*DRCMRM*). The query word(s) is used to generate a set of Blob probabilities from the joint distribution of blobs and words. This vector of Blob probabilities is compared with the vector of blobs for each test image using Kullback-Liebler (KL) divergence, and the resulting KL distance is used to rank the images.

Given a query $Q = w_1...w_k$ and the image $I = \{b_1...b_m\}$, it is supposed the existence of an underlying relevance model $P(.|Q)$ such that the query itself is a random sample from that model. It is also assumed that images relevant to Q are random samples from $P(.|Q)$. The query is converted into the language of blobs, and the probability of observing a given Blob b from the query model can be expressed in terms of the joint probability of observing b from the same distribution as the query words $w_1 \ldots w_k$ [28]:

$$P(b|Q) \approx P(b|w_1 \ldots w_k) = \frac{P(b, w_1 \ldots w_k)}{P(w_1 \ldots w_k)} \tag{6.2}$$

$$P(b, w_1, \ldots, w_k) = \sum_{J \in T} P(J)P(b|J) \prod_{i=1}^{k} P(w_i|J) \tag{6.3}$$

Based on this approach, images are ranked according to the negative Kullback-Liebler divergence between the query model $P(.|Q)$ and the image model $P(.|I)$ [28]:

$$-\operatorname{KL}(Q|I) = \sum_{b \in B} P(b|Q) \log \frac{P(b|I)}{P(b|Q)} \tag{6.4}$$

where $P(b|Q)$ is estimated using Eqs. 6.2 and 6.3, and $P(b|I)$ is estimated using Eq. 5.4 of CMRM. After the negative value of the divergence is calculated for each image, the first n images having the smallest values are kept.

6.3 Experimental Results

The evaluation was made on a database containing a number of 2,000 medical images with queries containing one, two, or three words in order to keep a good precision. After computing the probability of each image relatively to the query Q, only the first n images are kept, n being a configurable parameter. For a given query Q, the relevant images are the ones that contain all query words in the manual annotation. For testing purposes, we have considered the value 10 for parameter n. Table 6.1 shows the details of the three subsets of our query set, along with average precision for the two retrieval models on each of the subset. The performance is generally higher for longer queries. It can be observed that the direct-retrieval cross-media relevance model (DRCMRM) outperforms the probabilistic annotation-based cross-media relevance model (PACMRM) on all query subsets.

Figure 6.1 presents some of the relevant images that were retrieved for the following one-word queries:

Table 6.1 Different query sets and the relative performance of the two retrieval models in terms of average precision

Query length	1 word	2 words	3 words
Number of queries	220	457	190
Relevant images	1,543	1,231	720
Average precision (PACMRM)	0.173	0.162	0.198
Average precision (DRCMRM)	0.197	0.175	0.216

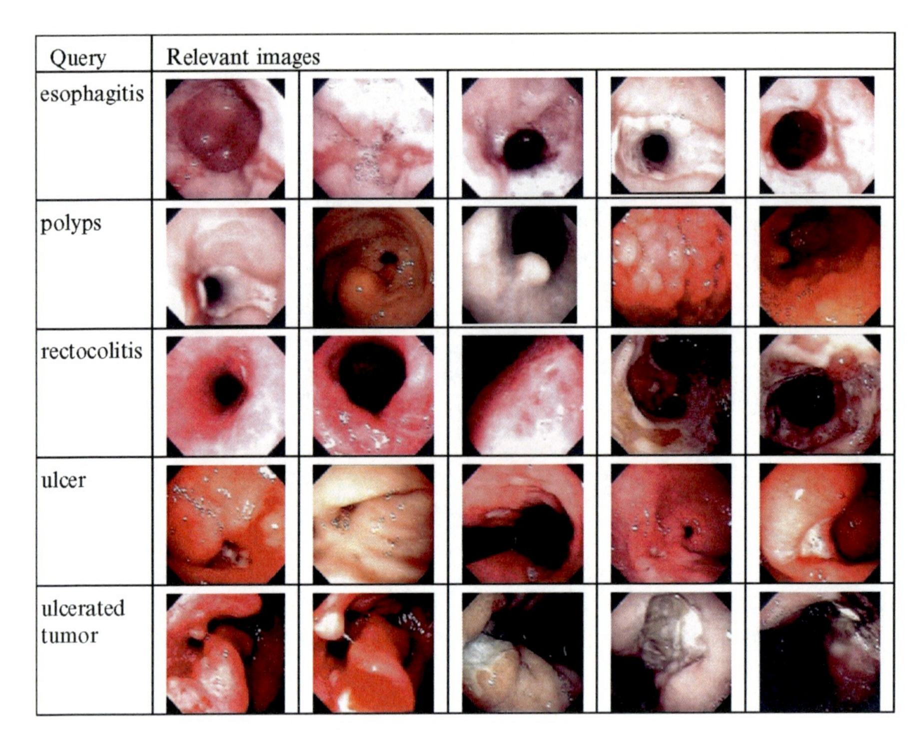

Fig. 6.1 Semantic-based image retrieval: experimental results

6.4 Conclusions

In this chapter, we have presented an overview of the existing methods that can be applied for the semantic-based image retrieval task and a description of two models (*PACMRM*, *DRCMRM*) provided by the CMRM model for the same task. We have used these models for the semantic retrieval task because they allow us to perform a ranked retrieval of images. Another reason was represented by the fact that we wanted to evaluate the CMRM model for image annotation and for semantic-based image retrieval.

The first model (*PCAMRM*) is using the entire probability distribution $P(.|I)$ to score images using a language-modeling approach. For a given query Q containing a list of words as input, it is provided as output a ranked list of images based on the probability computed for each image. The second model (*DRCMRM*) converts the query Q into the language of blobs. Using this approach, it is possible to directly retrieve images from the collection C by measuring how similar they are to the Blob representation of the query. Images are ranked according to the negative Kullback-Liebler divergence computed between the query model and the image model. The difference between the approaches used by the two models has shown that the second model produces better results in terms of precision. The experimental results made on queries with one, two, or three words have shown that the average precision has a better value for the second model.

In the future work, we intend to make a comparison between the two models mentioned above and other existing models for semantic-based image retrieval that are providing a ranked list of images. The database of medical images will be extended up to 10,000 medical images, and more detailed experiments will be performed.

References

1. Zhang YJ (2007) Semantic-based visual information retrieval. IRM Press, Hershey
2. Smeulders AWM, Worring M, Santini S, Gupta A, Jain R (2000) Content-based image retrieval at the end of the early years. IEEE Trans Pattern Anal Mach Intell 22(12):1349–1380
3. Zhang YJ (2007) Chapter I: Toward high-level visual information retrieval. In: Zhang Y-J (ed) Semantic-based visual information retrieval. IRM Press, Hershey
4. Chang SF, Chen W, Meng HJ, Sundaram H, Zhong D (1998) A fully automated content-based video search engine supporting spatiotemporal queries. IEEE CSVT 8(5):602–615
5. Naphade MR, Huang TS (2002) Extracting semantics from audiovisual content: The final frontier in multimedia retrieval. IEEE NN 13(4):793–810
6. Xu Y, Zhang YJ (2003) Semantic retrieval based on feature element constructional model and bias competition mechanism. SPIE 5021:77–88
7. Hanjalic A (2001) Video and image retrieval beyond the cognitive level: The needs and possibilities. SPIE 4315:130–140
8. Dasiopoulou S, Doulaverakis C, Mezaris V, Kompatsiaris I, Strintzis MG (2007) Chapter X: An ontology-based framework for semantic image analysis and retrieval. In: Zhang Y-J (ed) Semantic-based visual information retrieval. IRM Press, Hershey
9. Sesame. http://www.openrdf.org/. Accessed 24 Aug 2011
10. Cheng SC, Chou TC, Yang CL et al (2005) A semantic learning for content-based image retrieval using analytical hierarchy process. Expert Syst Appl 28(3):495–505
11. Schreiber A, Dubbeldam B, Wielemaker J, Wielinga BJ (2001) IEEE Intell Syst 16(3):66–74
12. Hollink L, Schreiber A, Wielemaker J, Wielinga B (2003) Semantic annotation of image collections. In: Proceedings of the workshop on knowledge markup and semantic annotation, Sanibel Island, 2003
13. Chen YX, Wang JZ, Krovetz R (2005) CLUE: cluster-based retrieval of images by unsupervised learning. IEEE IP 14(8):1187–1201
14. Reidsma D, Kuper J, Declerck T, Saggion H, Cunningham H (2003) Cross document annotation for multimedia retrieval. In: Proceedings of the 10th conference of the European chapter of the association for computational linguistics (EACL), Budapest, 2003
15. Lim JH, Jin JS (2005) Combining intra-image and inter-class semantics for consumer image retrieval. Pattern Recognit 38(6):847–864
16. Cristianini N, Shawe-Taylor J (2000) An introduction to support vector machines and other kernel-based learning methods. Cambridge University Press, New York
17. Thomure M (2004) Toward semantic image retrieval. Portland State University
18. Mitchell M, Hofstadter DR (1990) The emergence of understanding in a computer model of concepts and analogy-making. Phys D Nonlinear Phenom 42(1–3):322–334
19. Vogel J, Schiele B (2006) Performance evaluation and optimization for content-based image retrieval. Pattern Recognit 39:897–909

20. Maillot N, Thonnat M, Hudelot C (2004) Ontology based object learning and recognition: application to image retrieval. In: Proceedings of the 16th IEEE international conference on tools with artificial intelligence (ICTAI '04), Boca Raton, 2004, pp 620–625
21. Celebi E, Alpkocak A (2005) Combining textual and visual clusters for semantic image retrieval and auto-annotation. In: Proceedings of the 2nd European workshop on the integration of knowledge, semantics and digital media technology, London, 2005, pp 219–225
22. Fazli Can, Esen A. Ozkarahan (1985) Concepts of the cover coefficient-based clustering methodology. In: SIGIR '85: proceedings of the 8th annual international ACM SIGIR conference on research and development in information retrieval, New York, 1985
23. Mezaris V, Kompatsiaris I, Strintzis MG (2003) An ontology approach to object-based image retrieval. In: Proceedings of the 2003 international conference on image processing, Barcelona, 2003, vol 2, pp 511–514
24. Yoon J, Jayant M (2001) Relevance feedback for semantics based image retrieval. In: Proceedings of the international conference on image processing, Thessaloniki, 2001
25. Zhang D, Islam MM, Lu G, Hou J (2009) Semantic image retrieval using region based inverted file. In: Digital image computing: techniques and applications (DICTA '09), Melbourne, 2009, pp 242–249
26. Zhang R, Zhang Z, Li M, Ma W-Y, Zhang HJ (2005) A probabilistic semantic model for image annotation and multi-modal image retrieval. In: Proceedings of the international conference on computer vision, Beijing, 2005
27. IRMA. http://irma-project.org/index_en.php. Accessed 24 Aug 2011
28. Jeon J, Lavrenko V, Manmatha R (2003) Automatic image annotation and retrieval using cross-media relevance models. In: Proceedings of ACM SIGIR international conference on research and development in information retrieval (SIGIR), Toronto, 2003, pp 119–126

Chapter 7
Object Oriented Medical Annotation System

7.1 Software System Architecture

For validating and evaluating our tasks, we have designed a system called MASOO that can be used for three distinct tasks:

(a) Automatic image annotation using the cross-media relevance model (CMRM)
(b) Semantic-based image retrieval using two methods exposed by the CMRM model
(c) Content-based image retrieval based on color and texture features

System's architecture based on client–server interactions is presented in Fig. 7.1.
The system contains two main components that are communicating based on the principles defined for the networking and out-of-band signaling interaction types:

(a) A client component being used for:

- Image segmentation
- Features extraction
- Semantic-based image retrieval
- Content-based image retrieval
- Sending the list of Region objects using the dbo Client Module to the db4o Server Module to perform the annotation process
- Retrieving using the dbo Client Module the list of n Word objects detected by the annotation process and provided by the db4o Server Module.

(b) A server component being used for:

- Importing MeSH content
- Performing the manually annotation of images
- Obtaining the list of Blob objects using the clustering module
- Performing an automatic image annotation

L. Stanescu et al., *Creating New Medical Ontologies for Image Annotation: A Case Study*, SpringerBriefs in Electrical and Computer Engineering,
DOI 10.1007/978-1-4614-1909-9_7,

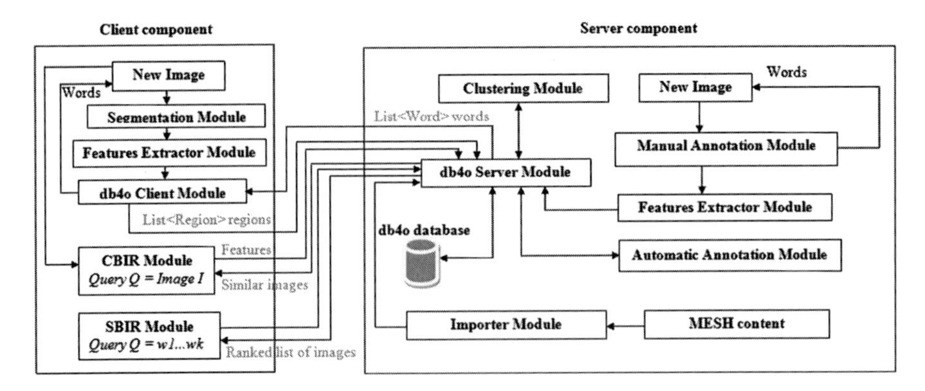

Fig. 7.1 System's architecture

The total number of distinct modules contained in this architecture is 10, and these will be described based on the flow (and in the logic order) required by the annotation process:

(a) db4o Server Module—this is the main module being used for storing and retrieving information in/from the database, for the annotation process, for content-based, and semantic-based image retrieval. All operations that are database related are passing through this module. It can be seen as a proxy for database access.
(b) Importer module—this module has as input the MeSH content which is offered as an .xml file named desc2010.xml (2010 version) containing the descriptors and a txt file named mtrees2010.txt containing the hierarchical structure of the descriptors. This module generates the ontology based on the information provided by MeSH. Each concept obtained based on the information provided by a descriptor will be represented as a Word object, and each hierarchical relationship between descriptors will be represented as a HierarchicalRelationship object between the two Word objects representing the parent–child relationship. At the end of this process, these objects are stored in the database, and the content of the ontology is exported as a Topic Map by generating an .xtm file using the xtm syntax. Using this approach, the content of the ontology can be seen in a graphical manner using a navigator that was designed for this purpose. After this module is applied, we have available the ontology that is needed for the annotation task.
(c) Manual annotation module—this module is used to obtain the training set of annotated images needed for the automatic annotation process. The specialist obtains a set of images collected from patients using an endoscope, and this set is placed in a specific disk location. Each image is manually segmented using a MATLAB tool named interactive segmentation and annotation tool (ISATOOL) which is presented in Fig. 7.2. ISATOOL allows the interactive segmentation of objects by drawing points around the desired object, while splines are used to join the marked points, which also produces fairly accurate

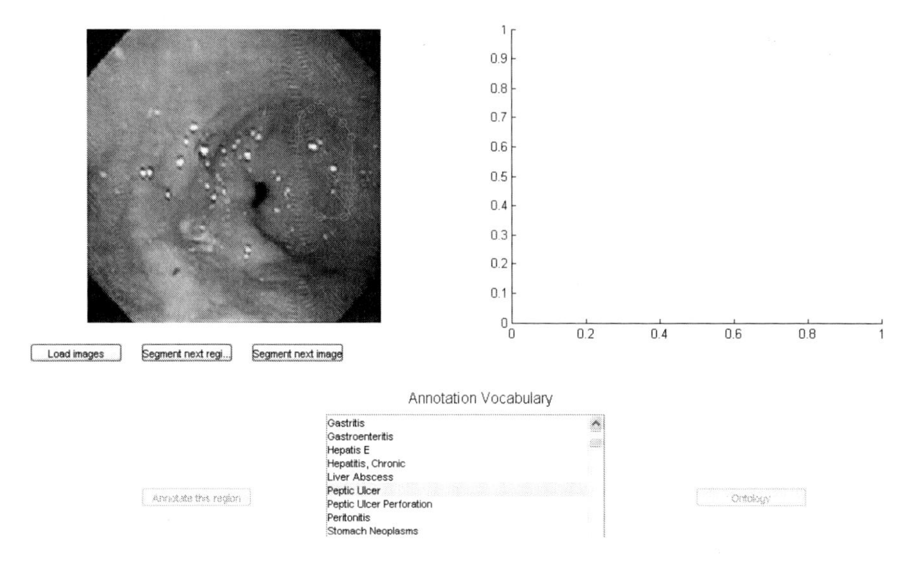

Fig. 7.2 ISATOOL interface

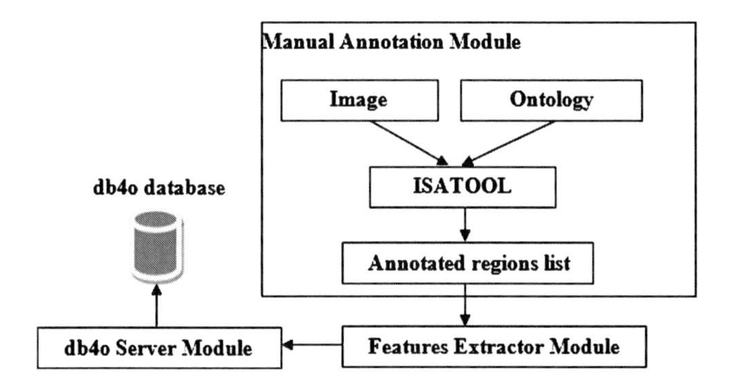

Fig. 7.3 Manual annotation process diagram

segmentation with much lower segmentation effort. Each region has associated a segmentation mask and a Word object from the ontology. This tool can also be used to extend the set of training images for the annotation model. After using this module, we have obtained a set of image regions that are manually annotated. Next, we need to apply a new module to extract the characteristics from each region. The diagram of the manual annotation process is depicted in Fig. 7.3.

(d) Segmentation module—this module performs the segmentation of an image into regions using our original segmentation algorithm based on a hexagonal structure that was described in a previous chapter. This module can be configured to segment all images from an existing images folder on the storage disk or a specific image given as input. The output is represented by a list of Region objects.

(e) Features extractor module—this module is receiving a list of Region objects and extracts feature vectors. For each region, a feature vector that contains visual information of the region such as color (color histogram with 166 bins in the HSV color space), texture (maximum probability, inverse difference moment, entropy, energy, contrast, correlation), position (minimum bounding rectangle), and shape (area, perimeter, convexity, compactness) is computed. The components of the feature vector are used to fill a FeaturesVector object that is set as a property of the corresponding Region object. In this moment, we have a training set of image regions available that are manually annotated and having associated a feature vector. Now, it is the time to cluster the regions in a number of clusters using the next module.

(f) Clustering module—we have used K-means algorithm with a fixed value of 500 (this means that 500 clusters will be created) to quantize the feature vectors obtained from the training set and to generate blobs (representing clusters of image regions). Each blob is represented as a Blob object. After the quantization, each image in the training set is represented as a set of Blob object identifiers. For each Blob object, a median feature vector and a list of words belonging to the test images that have that blob in their representation are computed. The values of the median feature vector are stored in a FeaturesVector object. The median feature vector is set as a value for the property called AverageFeaturesVector of the corresponding Blob object. Each word from the detected list is represented as a Word object. The AverageFeaturesVector is needed because the annotation algorithm applied for a new image requires the identification of the list of Blob objects that are appropriate (more closer in the features space) for image regions. After using this module, we have available 500 blobs of image regions, and from this moment, we have the elements required by the annotation model.

(g) Automatic annotation module—this module is used to annotate a new image. When a new image needs to be annotated, this module receives as input from the db4o Server Module, the list of regions belonging to the new image. After that, the list of Word objects is computed by applying the object-oriented approach of the CMRM model. The list of words represents the output of this module and is sent back to the db4o Sever Module. Generally speaking, an annotation request will come from the module called db4o Client Module through db4o Server Module which behaves as an intermediate. The list of Word objects will be sent back as a response by the db4o Server Module to the db4o Client Module. The annotation process that is performed by the automatic annotation module will be summarized shortly. For each Region object received in the input, the Blob object which is closest to it in the cluster space is assigned. The assigned Blob object has the minimum value of the Euclidian distance computed between the AverageFeaturesVector of that Blob object and the FeaturesVector object of the Region object. In this way, the new image will be represented by a set of Blob object identifiers. Having the set of Blob objects and for each Blob having a list of Word objects, a list of potential Word objects that can be assigned to the image is determined.

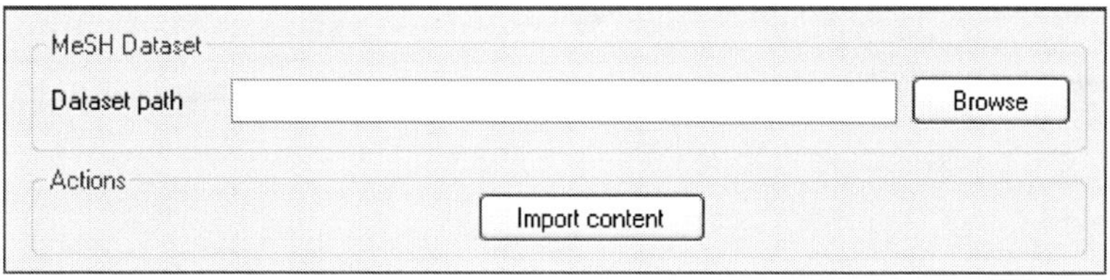

Fig. 7.4 Options available for importing MeSH dataset

For each Word, the probability to be assigned to the image is computed. The list containing probability values is sorted in a descending order, and after that, the set of top n (configurable value) words having high probability value will be used to annotate the image.

(h) db4o Client Module—this module is used to send to the db4o Server Module a list of Region objects representing the regions of the image that should be annotated. The list of Word objects received back as the result of the annotation task is assigned to the image.

(i) Content-based image retrieval (CBIR) module—this module extracts a features vector from the image given as input, and then, it sends it to the db4o Server Module. This module then computes the similarity distance between the feature vector received belonging to the analyzed image and the existing feature vectors in the database. When this process is completed, it returns back a list of similar images having the value of the computed distance smaller than a threshold value which is configurable.

(j) Semantic-based image retrieval (SBIR) module—this module sends a list of Word objects given as query to the db4o Server Module. This module is capable of using the two types of semantic-based image retrieval provided by CMRM against a query $Q = w_1 \ldots w_k$. After performing the required computation, the ranked list of n images containing objects described by the words $w_1 \ldots w_k$ is returned back as a result.

The operations that can be performed using the GUI of the system are:

(a) Importing the content of the MeSH dataset—the dataset contains a number of 5,000 images that are used as a training set for the annotation model. Each image was manually segmented, and each region has assigned a concept from the ontology. Several files containing the features extracted from regions are made available and are used to retrieve and store the values in the database. The features are used by the clustering algorithm to compute the blobs. The content of the dataset is imported using the options shown in Fig. 7.4.

(b) Obtaining clusters and filtering—having available in the database the features extracted from regions, it can be applied the K-means algorithm to obtain the list of blobs (clusters of regions). We have used a number of 500 clusters for our dataset. After the clustering process is completed, the regions contained in each cluster can be seen after performing a filtering by cluster number using the options provided in Fig. 7.5. This option is useful to validate the result of the clustering operation and to have an overview of what regions are contained in each cluster.

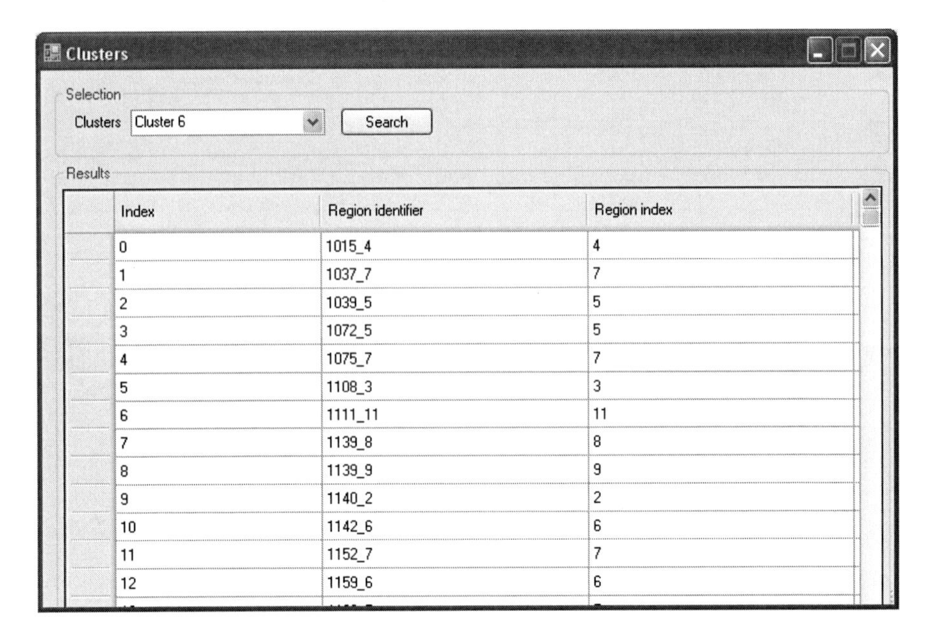

Index	Region identifier	Region index
0	1015_4	4
1	1037_7	7
2	1039_5	5
3	1072_5	5
4	1075_7	7
5	1108_3	3
6	1111_11	11
7	1139_8	8
8	1139_9	9
9	1140_2	2
10	1142_6	6
11	1152_7	7
12	1159_6	6

Fig. 7.5 Options available for viewing clusters content

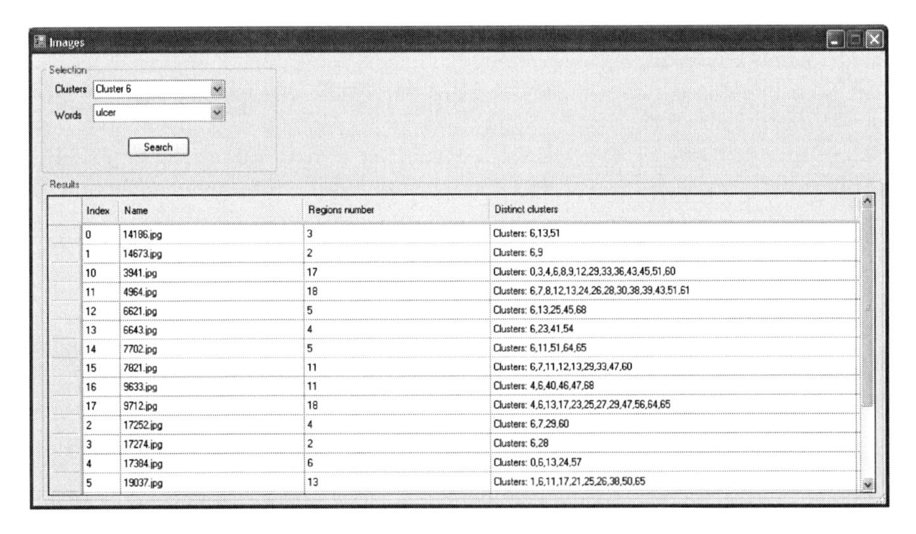

Index	Name	Regions number	Distinct clusters
0	14186.jpg	3	Clusters: 6,13,51
1	14673.jpg	2	Clusters: 6,9
10	3941.jpg	17	Clusters: 0,3,4,6,8,9,12,29,33,36,43,45,51,60
11	4964.jpg	18	Clusters: 6,7,8,12,13,24,26,28,30,38,39,43,51,61
12	6621.jpg	5	Clusters: 6,13,25,45,68
13	6643.jpg	4	Clusters: 6,23,41,54
14	7702.jpg	5	Clusters: 6,11,51,64,65
15	7821.jpg	11	Clusters: 6,7,11,12,13,29,33,47,60
16	9633.jpg	11	Clusters: 4,6,40,46,47,68
17	9712.jpg	18	Clusters: 4,6,13,17,23,25,27,29,47,56,64,65
2	17252.jpg	4	Clusters: 6,7,29,60
3	17274.jpg	2	Clusters: 6,28
4	17384.jpg	6	Clusters: 0,6,13,24,57
5	19037.jpg	13	Clusters: 1,6,11,17,21,25,26,38,50,65

Fig. 7.6 Filtering images using the cluster number and/or a word

(c) Filtering images—filtering of images can be performed by specifying the cluster number and/or a word. It can be observed that for each image, it is shown the number of regions and the list of blobs assigned to that image. The list of clusters contains the blobs identifiers (Fig. 7.6).

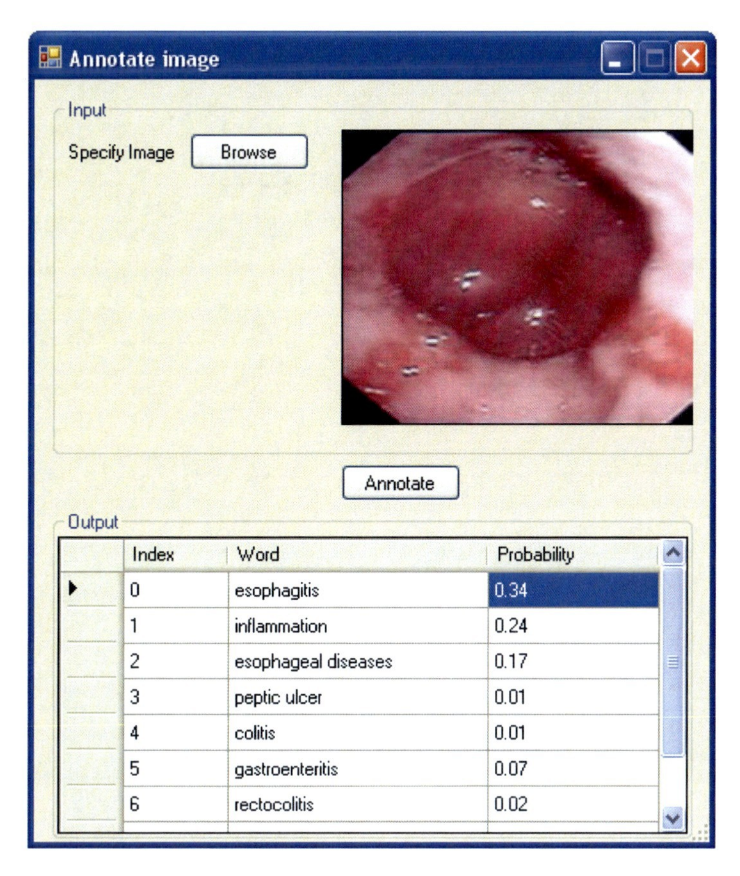

Fig. 7.7 Image annotation interface

Using this screen, the information (image name, number of regions, blobs assigned) about images from the database or which are the images annotated with a specific word can be seen.

(a) Image annotation—the probability of each word to be associated with that image is calculated by giving a test image. The list containing the probabilities for all words is sorted in a descending order, and only the top *n* words are used to annotate the image. This process is depicted in Fig. 7.7 where an image having the esophagitis diagnostic can be annotated with the first three words having the highest probabilities.
(b) Semantic-based image retrieval—using the methods provided by CMRM for semantic-based image retrieval and a query containing a list of words, a semantic-based image retrieval operation can be performed. The user has the possibility to select the list of words, and for each image in the dataset, the probability to be relevant for that query is computed. Only images that contain all query words are considered relevant. After the probability is calculated for

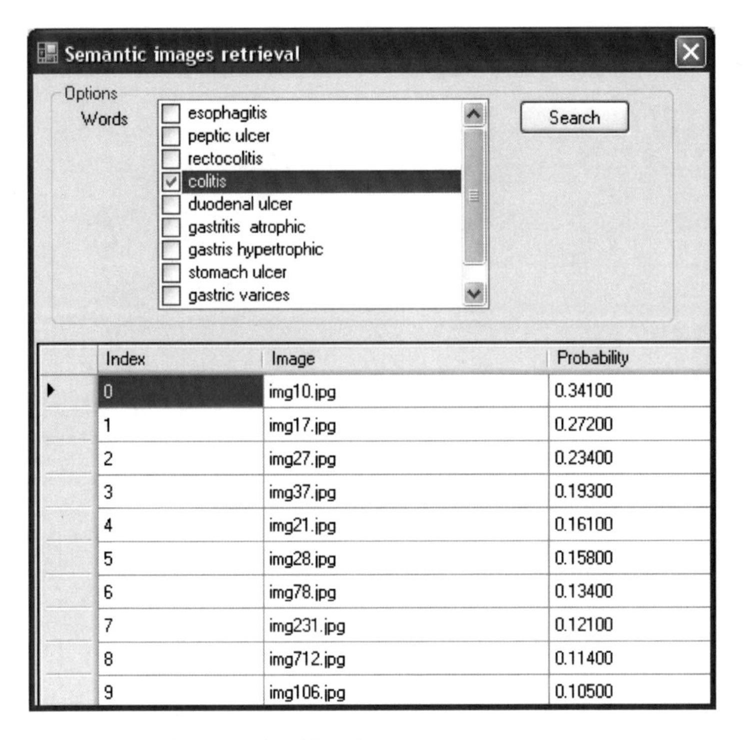

Fig. 7.8 Semantic-based image retrieval interface

each image, the list of all probabilities is sorted in a descending order. The first n images having higher probabilities are kept. This operation is depicted in Fig. 7.8.

(c) Content-based image retrieval—the user can specify the query image that will be used for image retrieval. From that image, a feature vector that is compared against the list of all feature vectors existing in the database is extracted. The comparison is based on the similarity distance computed between vectors. The first n images having the lowest distance will be included in the result. This operation is depicted in Fig. 7.9 where it is given an example for an image with ulcer diagnostic.

7.2 Conclusions

We have presented our system created for evaluating the performance of the annotation and retrieval (semantic-based and content-based) tasks. Our system provides support for all steps that are required for evaluating the tasks mentioned

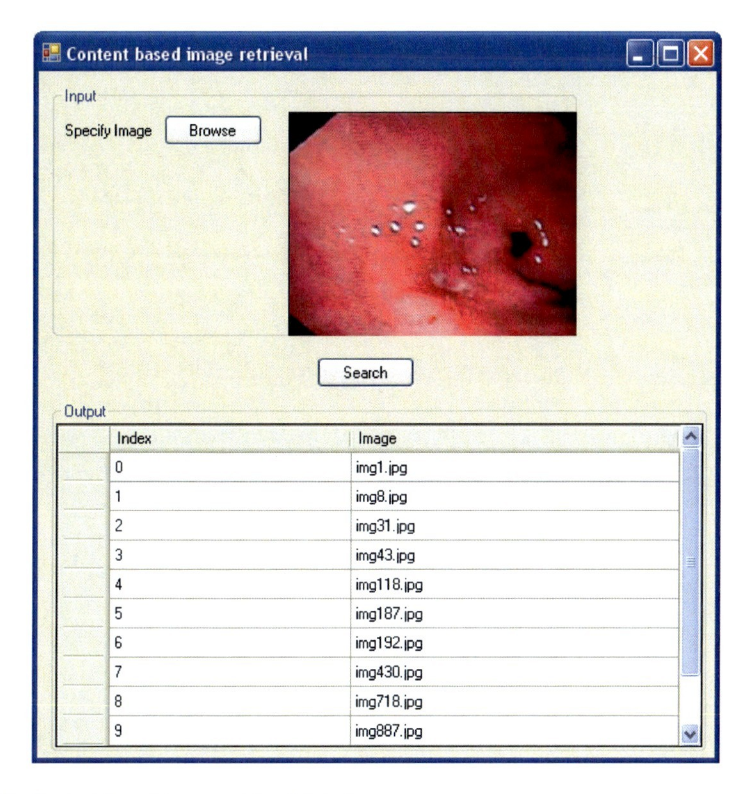

Fig. 7.9 Content-based image retrieval interface

above, starting with data import, knowledge storage and representation, knowledge presentation, and means for tasks evaluation. GUIs are made available by the system to present the information in a user-friendly manner and to simplify the steps that should be applied to obtain what is intended.

In this moment, the system is tested by the medical specialists from the Romanian University hospital "Filantropia" on medical images that represent the digestive tract diseases. The feedback that will be received about the usability and the performance results will be taken into account for further improvements. GUIs will be updated based on their feedback in order to increase the usability. The first report that was received and containing the results obtained after using the system in the initial phase was promising.

In the near future, it is expected that this system will be capable enough of providing information about an automated image diagnostic regarding the digestive tract diseases.